Non-Sterile Compounding for Pharmacy Technicians

Notice

Non-Sterile Compounding for Pharmacy Technicians

Training and Review for Certification

Denise Propes, CPhT

Senior and Lead Technician
University of Michigan Hospital
and Health Systems Research Pharmacy
(Investigational Drug Service)
Ann Arbor, Michigan

Etta Johnson, CPhT

Professional Services Support
Fagron, Inc.
St. Paul, Minnesota

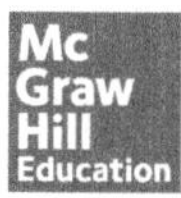

New York Chicago San Francisco Athens London Madrid
Mexico City Milan New Delhi Singapore Sydney Toronto

Non-Sterile Compounding for Pharmacy Technicians: Training and Review for Certification

1 2 3 4 5 6 7 8 9 0 CTP/CTP 19 18 17 16 15 14

ISBN 978-0-07-182988-5
MHID 0-07-182988-1

This book was set in Minion by Cenveo® Publisher Services.
The editors were Michael Weitz and Peter J. Boyle.
The production supervisor was Catherine H. Saggese.
Project management was provided by Anupriya Tyagi, Cenveo Publisher Services.
The designer was Elise Lansdon; the cover designer was Thomas DePierro.
China Translation & Printing Services, Ltd., was printer and binder.

This book is printed on acid-free paper.

This book is dedicated to all the pharmacists and technicians who provide compounding services to improve the quality of life of their patients every day.

Etta and Denise

To my husband Robert and my family, thank you for all your love and support.

To all my coworkers in the University of Michigan Research Pharmacy, thank you for your friendship and encouragement.

Denise Propes

To the wise and caring pharmacists who taught me to compound.

To my mother Jane, whose hospice-managed death in 1996 showed me the actual value of what I had learned.

Etta L. Johnson

Contents

Preface

The art of pharmacy compounding can be traced back thousands of years. Today's compounding pharmacy combines this ancient art with the latest advances in medical science and modern technology. A pharmacy technician who has acquired the knowledge and skills needed to work in this specialized pharmacy practice sector has an opportunity to enhance the quality of patient care while increasing his or her own marketability and career opportunities.

As pharmacy technicians and educators, we have designed *Non-Sterile Compounding for Pharmacy Technicians: Training and Review for Certification* in a friendly, casual format intended to promote and maintain the reader's interest in this unique and creative segment of pharmacy. This text explains in detail the tools, equipment, and documents necessary to ensure the quality preparation of compounded pharmaceuticals. It includes easy-to-follow, step by step procedures for preparing liquid, solid, and semisolid compounded dosage forms. Each chapter features PTCB formatted review questions, calculation exercises designed to reinforce concepts, and discussion topics to promote creative thinking and student involvement.

Non-Sterile Compounding for Pharmacy Technicians includes all the concepts and processes necessary to prepare the student, novice, or seasoned pharmacy technician with the tools and knowledge necessary either to enter this growing pharmacy sector or enhance and refresh the skills they already possess in order to be successful in any non-sterile compounding practice environment.

Acknowledgments

Administrative assistance and support: James W. Propes and Lillian S. Propes.

Reviewer and Contributor: Kristy Malacos, MS, CPhT, Pharmacy Administrator, Magruder Hospital, Pharmacy Systems, Inc., Port Clinton, Ohio.

A special thanks to Michael Weitz, Peter Boyle, and all the McGraw-Hill Education staff who assisted in the development and design of this project.

CHAPTER 1

The Definition of Compounding

INTRODUCTION

The art of pharmacy compounding can be traced back thousands of years. Today's compounding pharmacy combines this ancient art with the latest in medical science and modern technology. A technician who has gained the knowledge and skills needed to work in this unique environment has an opportunity to make great contributions to patient **compliance** and outcomes. Compounding can be thought of in two parts: first, the importance of compounding to health care in the modern world and second, the standard of practice including the regulations that must be followed to ensure the safety of the compounded preparation, and thus the safety of the patient.

LEARNING OBJECTIVES

- Understand the definition of pharmacy compounding and its benefits.
- Understand the difference between manufacturing and compounding processes.
- Understand the purpose of non-sterile compounding.
- Understand USP/NF Chapter <795> compounding guidelines.
- Understand regulations and laws pertaining to compounding.
- Understand and use non-sterile compounding resources.

KEY TERMS

CE: Continuing education

Compliance: To fulfill stated requirements or regulations

Compound: Any material consisting of more than one substance, either occurring in nature or created synthetically in a laboratory

Compounded medication: A medication that is not available as a manufactured product and is prepared by a pharmacist to be provided to a particular patient based on the written order of a licensed prescriber and is not available as a manufactured product

Drug monograph: A complete description of a specific drug

Excipient: An inactive substance or "filler" used in combination with an active medication or substance

Formulation: Complete written, documented instruction on how to prepare a particular compounded medication

Prescription: An instruction from a licensed prescriber, to a registered pharmacist to provide a necessary medication to a patient

PURPOSE

The purpose of compounding is simple: *find and provide ways to help patients get the medications they require.* The proper practice of compounding can solve problems that interfere with compliance within a prescribed course of drug therapy and help assist in positive patient outcomes.

For example, if a child needs a medication that is only available in capsule form, but is incapable of swallowing a capsule, a compounded oral liquid containing the proper amount of drug per dose may be compounded. Additionally, a compounded transdermal medication may be used to improve the quality of life for patients by allowing them to avoid invasive dosage forms such as injections or intravenous therapy. Also, a **compounded medication** may be the only way to provide a patient with the proper medication in cases where the commercially manufactured product contains an ingredient to which they experience an adverse reaction. A common example would be the patient who experiences severe lactose intolerance but requires medication which is only available in a capsule that contains lactose as the filler. Short-term use of the manufactured capsule may not cause problems, but long-term use could provide a problem with compliance. Even if the patient only *perceives* that the small amount of lactose in a capsule will make them uncomfortable, targets for clinical outcomes can be affected in a negative way.

Although some formulas may be complex, compounding can really be as simple as adding a flavoring to a liquid medication. This can truly assist in helping to achieve compliance, especially for pediatric patients. A capsule containing several medications prepared for a patient who has difficulty swallowing is also considered a compounded medication. Compounded medications provide a vast array of options that improve patient outcomes and compliance to drug regimens.

Non-sterile compounding in the pharmacy provides a valuable contribution to patient care and quality of life. Certified pharmacy technicians assist in the preparation of compounded medications in pharmacies across the United States and around the world. Pharmacy technicians who are properly trained in compounding can make a valuable contribution to a patient's well-being and the health care industry.

Pharmacy compounding refers to incorporation of a drug into a suitable dosage form to provide a medication that is not available in a manufactured product in a proper dose or form for a particular patient.

DEFINITION

In pharmaceutical terminology a **compound** is any material consisting of more than one substance. For example, sodium is *not* a compound. Sodium phosphate *is* a compound. Cocoa Butter USP is not a compound; it is just pure cocoa butter. In this sense, a compound either occurs in nature or is created synthetically in a laboratory. Many such compounds are manufactured to meet the common medication needs of patients.

By definition a compounded medication *is* a **prescription** drug. In the United States, a prescription is an instruction from a licensed prescriber to a registered pharmacist to provide necessary medication to a patient. A compounded medication allows the patient to obtain the exact dose, in the best form to help them follow the therapy determined by the prescriber.

In the current written instructions for enforcement, a compounded medication is considered a *new drug* by the US Food and Drug Administration (FDA); however, traditional compounding is performed every day because sometimes a compounded medication is the only way to deliver the drug therapy a patient requires. Compounding provides necessary, prescribed medications for *specific patients.* Any registered pharmacist in the United States may compound a medication for a specific patient on the order of a licensed prescriber.

HISTORY

Compounding pharmaceuticals is as old as the art of medicine. One of the earliest records of compounding was the Ebers papyrus (named after George Ebers, who discovered it) that dates to 1500 BC (Figure 1-1). It contains over 800 compounded remedies for common and advanced illnesses. The first known pharmacy was established in Baghdad in 754. In 869 a

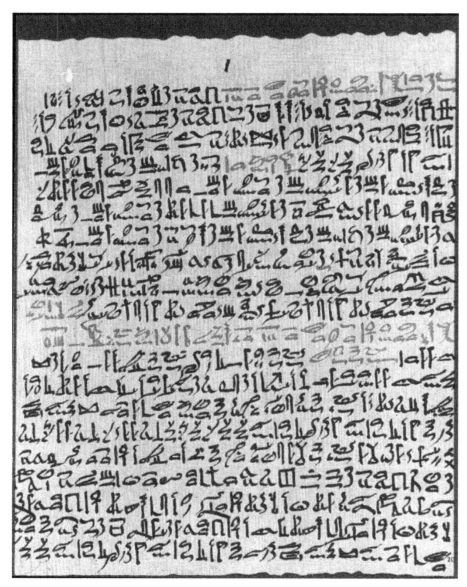

FIGURE 1-1 Ebers papyrus. (Source: *U.S. National Medical Library, National Institutes of Health, Washington, DC.*)

physician known as Sabur Ibn Sahl was the first to initiate and write an encyclopedia for drugs and remedies. Claudius Galenus or Galen made great contributions to the field of pharmacy compounding. He was a prominent Roman physician who ministered to many Roman emperors. The principles of compounding he established were used for over 1500 years. Many of the procedures he created are similar to those used in compounding pharmacies today.

In the 13th century, Frederick II, an Emperor in Germany and the King of Sicily, issued a decree separating the apothecary profession from the physician, but during Medieval times priests often ministered to the poor using herbal compounds. The first pharmacy in Europe was established in Germany in 1241 and is still in existence today.

Compounding in the United States can be traced back almost to the country's beginning. In early days, there were no large manufacturing facilities for drugs, so all pharmacies were compounding pharmacies. As late as the 1940s almost half the medications prescribed by doctors were compounds. Today compounded medications account for about 3% of the prescribed medications in the United States each year.

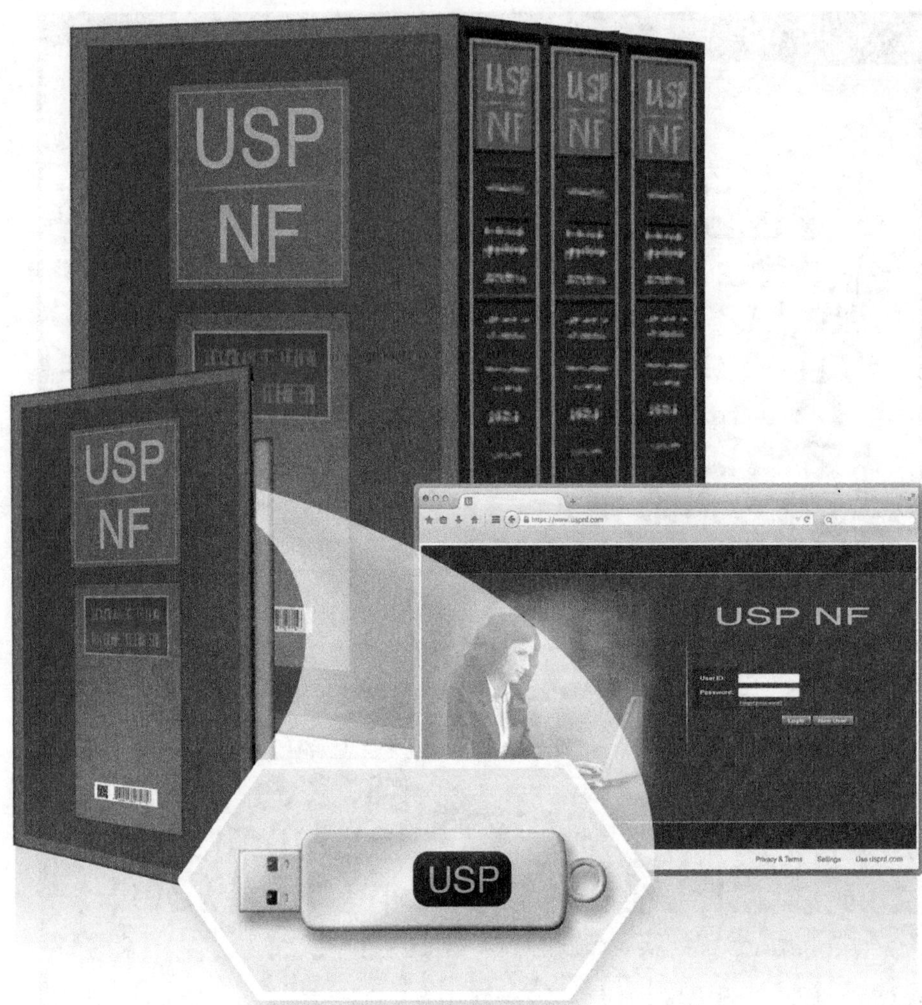

FIGURE 1-2 United States Pharmacopeia/National Formulary (USP/NF) (www.uspnf.com). *(Reproduced with permission from United States Pharmacopeial Convention, Rockville, MD.)*

USP/NF

The regulations that define pharmacy compounding are established by the *United States Pharmacopeia/National Formulary* (USP/NF) (Figure 1-2). The USP/NF was first published in 1820 and it was, and still is, prepared and modified by a group of individuals chosen to maintain the highest standards of pharmacy practice in the United States. Throughout its history, the USP committee has established standards that take into consideration the needs of patients, prescribers, and pharmacists. The publication produced by this body guides *all* manufacturing of drugs products—from the type of materials that may be used in packaging, to label requirements, package inserts. The USP/NF contains **drug monographs** (full descriptions) of all active and **excipient** ingredients that may be contained in medications used in the United States. In addition, these regulations include two specific chapters on pharmacy compounding: USP/NF Chapter ⟨795⟩ establishes rules for compounded non-sterile medications, and USP Chapter ⟨797⟩ establishes the rules for sterile compounding.

USP/NF Chapter <795> establishes the rules for preparation of non-sterile compounded medications.

Like all rules and regulations, the interpretation of what defines proper compounding can sometimes vary. Throughout your career as a certified pharmacy technician, you will encounter changes in what is allowed, what will be covered by insurance, and what is "popular" in pharmacy compounding. Regardless of the ongoing changes, certain basic definitions and rules will always apply.

USP/NF CHAPTER <795>

Rules developed by the USP/NF Committees are approved and made regulation (codified) by the US Congress. Chapter ⟨795⟩ of the USP/NF defines all non-sterile compounding rules and regulations. Several sections of this chapter give specific instructions on how compounding must be performed. This includes equipment that must be on hand in the compounding area, cleaning procedures, and documentation of the **formulation** and materials used in each particular compounded preparation.

It is the responsibility of the pharmacist to ensure that the rules are understood and followed by their staff. The rules of compounding are a work-in-progress, and the compounding technician can contribute to the practice by being aware of the regulations and alert to ongoing changes.

Although the regulations are established at the federal level, they are enforced at the state level by the state board of pharmacy. *It is the state board of pharmacy, not the federal government, that regulates pharmacy compounding within each state.* The USP/NF and FDA establish the rules. The state board of pharmacy adopts or modifies these rules to make them specific to the needs of the citizens of that state and enforces the regulations in pharmacies licensed by the state.

The state boards of pharmacy inspect and evaluate the pharmacy practice and its compounding activities. Because they enforce the rules, they have the best answer to any legal or regulatory question.

Whenever there is a question about a rule of compounding, the state board of pharmacy should be consulted.

Recently, a new body has been established to certify that pharmacies that practice traditional compounding are practicing within the regulations and up to the highest standards. Pharmacy organizations such as American Society of Health System Pharmacists (ASHP) and the International Academy of Compounding Pharmacists (IACP) in conjunction with State Boards of pharmacy and USP have come together to create a Pharmacy Compounding Accreditation Board (PCAB), although board certification is not yet required by any state or by the USP/NF regulations. Only about 150 pharmacies have achieved this "official" board certification, but every practice is expected to follow the regulations that apply to the compounded medications that are prepared.

MANUFACTURING VERSUS COMPOUNDING

Manufactured Drugs

The majority of drugs dispensed in pharmacies in the United States are manufactured drugs that have been evaluated by the FDA as safe and effective. Pharmaceutical manufacturers spend millions of dollars on research and development before a new drug is released to the market. Each drug goes through a series of clinical trials to test safety and efficacy on a small but significant number of patients. New drugs are intended to treat a specific indication. A retail pharmacy, hospital, home health care pharmacy, or skilled nursing facility purchases these manufactured drugs from a pharmaceutical wholesaler for resale or distribution to their patients. All manufacturers are inspected regularly by the FDA.

Compounded Drugs

Compounded medications are always prescription medications. They are prepared only on the written order of a licensed prescriber. Compounded medications provide an option for the patient who cannot fully benefit from the commercial dose or dosage form. A compounded medication should never be made to duplicate an available manufactured product unless the commercial product is unavailable.

If the exact medication the patient requires is available in a manufactured product, the compounder may *not* compound a duplication of that medication for *any reason*.

For example, a prescriber might write a prescription for a compounded medication because they know the patient cannot afford to purchase the manufactured product. In this case the pharmacist must explain that they cannot duplicate a commercially available product simply for the purpose of saving the patient money. However, if the manufactured medication contains an ingredient which is harmful to the patient, a compounded medication could be allowed.

The distinction between compounding and manufacturing is extremely important and also somewhat confusing. The technician is not responsible for this distinction, but the best question to ask if you are confused between compounding and manufacturing is: Who collected payment? Commercial drug manufacturers do not collect payment from any patient, insurance company, or health management organization. Manufacturers generally are paid by wholesale distributors. Unlike manufacturers, or wholesale distributors, pharmacies *do* collect payment from the patient and/or a third party (insurance provider).

Providing compounded medications to a physician who then dispenses and collects payment from a patient or their agent would be *manufacturing for resale* rather than compounding. A compounding pharmacy must not manufacture; they must limit themselves to filling prescriptions.

Making this distinction and following the rules are crucial to the protection of patient health and of the practice of compounding.

RESOURCES

Compounding uses an abundance of resources. Some are needed to assist the compounding pharmacist and their staff in basic knowledge such as calculations and compounding techniques. Other resources help determine the best method of delivering a certain medication to the patient. Other resources provide documented formulations.

Perhaps the most valuable single book used as a reference in a compounding pharmacy practice is *Trissel's Stability of Compounded Formulations* (Figure 1-3). Through five editions, it is a resource widely used to determine proper formulation and to document stability information as it relates to compounded preparations. *Martindale: The Complete Drug Reference* and *Remington: The Science and Practice of Pharmacy* contain monographs with very detailed information regarding the use of specific drugs. These complete monographs contain sections on how the drug is processed within the body and how it is administered, as well as contraindications and dangerous drug interactions.

Other compounding resources include pharmacy technician organizations such as the National Pharmacy Technician Association (NPTA) and the American Association of Pharmacy Technicians (AAPT), which strive to provide a wide variety of **continuing education (CE)** and are frequently adding compounding topics to their meeting agendas and CE libraries. There are also local and state pharmacy associations, online and written pharmacy journals, chemical and compounding trade organizations and suppliers who offer educational programs and updates on compounding rules. As your interest in becoming a compounding technician expands, so should your resources; attend a pharmacy convention (there are some just for compounding), use the Internet to find the latest news and information, attend a live CE, or find a written CE that pertains to compounding.

CONCLUSION

So again, the definition of compounding for our purposes is: the preparation by a registered pharmacist of a medication prescribed for a specific patient by a licensed prescriber. This specialized practice is allowed for the following reasons:

1. The best therapy for the patient requires a different dosage form than is provided by a manufactured product.
2. The best therapy for the patient requires a different concentration of the active drug than can be provided by a manufactured medication.

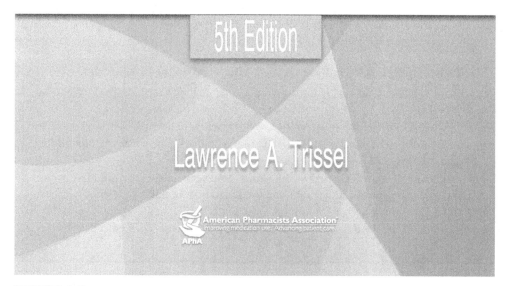

FIGURE 1-3 Trissel's Stability of Compounded Formulations. *(Reproduced with permission from the American Pharmacists Association, Washington, DC.)*

3. The manufactured product available contains an ingredient that the patient cannot tolerate.
4. The manufactured medication that has been prescribed is temporarily unavailable in its manufactured form, or has been discontinued for some reason other than safety or efficacy.
5. Compliance and patient outcomes would be improved by the combination of two or more drugs into one dosage form.

Now we will roll up our sleeves and begin to look into the actual work of compounding. In the following chapters we discuss the general layout of a pharmacy compounding area, the tools that are available to accomplish the task of compounding, and the fundamental process that must be in place to provide patients with the medications they require. Compounding is problem solving. Let's learn together how to identify and solve problems through pharmacy compounding.

CHAPTER SUMMARY

- The purpose of compounding is to find and provide ways to help patients get the medications they require.
- A compounded medication allows the patient to obtain the exact dose, in the best form to follow the therapy determined by their physician.
- Any registered pharmacist in the United States may compound a medication for a specific patient on the order of a licensed prescriber.
- A compound is any material consisting of more than one substance.
- A compounded medication is a prescription drug, prescribed and prepared for a specific patient.
- Before there were large manufacturing facilities for drugs, all pharmacies were compounding pharmacies.
- The regulations that define pharmacy compounding are established by the United States Pharmacopeia/National Formulary (USP/NF).
- The USP/NF contains monographs (full descriptions) of all active and excipient ingredients that may be contained in medications used in the United States.
- USP/NF Chapter ⟨795⟩ establishes the rules for preparation of non-sterile compounded medications.
- USP Chapter ⟨797⟩ establishes rules for compounded sterile medications.
- State Boards of Pharmacy regulates and enforces rules for pharmacy compounding within each state.
- Manufactured drugs dispensed in the United States are deemed by the FDA as safe and effective for specific indications and used in a large number of patients.
- If the exact medication a patient requires is available as a manufactured product, a compounded medication which duplicates that manufactured medication cannot be made.

PTCB Review Questions

Select the correct answer to the following multiple choice questions.

1. The regulations that define pharmacy compounding are established by
   A. ASHP
   B. Compounding pharmacies
   C. USP/NF
   D. IACP
2. Compounding rules are enforced by which agency within the state?
   A. USP
   B. IACP
   C. State board of pharmacy
   D. FDA

3. Who can compound prescription medications?
   A. Only a pharmacist licensed with a compounding certification.
   B. Any registered pharmacist in the United States.
   C. A pharmacy technician under the supervision of a licensed pharmacist.
   D. B and C.
4. Non-sterile compounding rules are established in a specific chapter in which publication?
   A. USP/NF
   B. State board of pharmacy
   C. FDA
   D. PTCB
5. A compound is defined as which of the following?
   A. A chemical
   B. A manufactured medication
   C. One ingredient
   D. Any material consisting of more than one substance
6. Compounding for patients is *not* allowed if the following situations exist.
   A. The doctor wants to save the patient some money.
   B. The physician asks.
   C. The same product is commercially available in the exact dosage form and strength.
   D. All of the above.
7. Which of the following statements are *true* regarding non-sterile compounding?
   A. A compounded medication is a prescription medication, prescribed and prepared for a specific patient.
   B. A pharmacist may compound a medication and sell it to a physician so that he can sell it to his patients.
   C. Compounding and manufacturing are the same things.
   D. None of the above.
8. Which publication is used to find information related to the stability of compounded preparations?
   A. USP/NF Chapter ⟨795⟩
   B. Pharmacy CEs
   C. *Trissel's Stability of Compounded Formulations*
   D. State board of pharmacy
9. Pharmacies can compound for the following reasons.
   A. To improve patient compliance to dosing regiments.
   B. Because the correct dosage is not commercially available.
   C. To save a patient money.
   D. Both A and B.
10. Choose the *false* statement as it pertains to non-sterile compounding.
    A. A patient can ask for a compounded medication in order to save money.
    B. A compounded prescription must be for a specific patient.
    C. The USP/NF contains full descriptions of all active and excipient ingredients that may be contained in medications used in the United States.
    D. Whenever there is a question about a rule of compounding, the state board of pharmacy should be consulted.

This chapter includes the following PTCE Blueprint Knowledge Areas

Section 3.0 Sterile and non-sterile compounding

Section 2.0-2.13 Professional standards regarding the roles and responsibilities of pharmacist, pharmacy technicians, and other pharmacy employees

This chapter meets the following ASHP goals and instructional objectives for Pharmacy Technician Training

OBJ 3.1 Explain how state laws and regulations determine what activities associated with preparing medications for distribution can be delegated by pharmacists to technicians.

OBJ 11.1 Follow established policies and procedures for monitoring the practice site and/or service area for compliance with federal, state, and local laws; regulations; and professional standards.

OBJ 22.1 Explain the benefits of membership in the range of local, state, and national pharmacy organizations.

OBJ 22.2 Describe the local, state, and national pharmacy organizations that offer value for the pharmacy technician.

OBJ 24.2 Discuss resources (eg, journals, newsletters, educational conferences) for staying current with advances in pharmacy practice (eg, automation, medication therapy, devices).

This chapter meets the following Ex-CPT Test Specifications

Section 1 A-3 Differentiate between tasks that may be performed by a pharmacy technician and those that must performed by a pharmacist.

Section 1 C-8 Comply with professional, state, and federal laws and regulations.

Section 3 B-5 Follow proper recordkeeping procedures pertaining to the pharmacy.

Section 3 D-1 Follow proper compounding procedures for non-sterile products.

Techs in Practice: Discussion Topics and Questions

What relatively recent events have brought pharmacy compounding to the attention of the American people?

1. Will these events change how compounding pharmacies and other health organizations that compound operate?
2. What kinds of things do you think will change?

SCENARIO 1

In 2009 a compounding pharmacy prepared an injectable (sterile) medication to be administered to polo ponies prior to an important tournament. Twenty-one horses died of a miscalculation of the dose provided. This activity made the national news for several consecutive days and caused a great outcry as well as criminal charges brought against the pharmacist. This affected all compounding practices because the word "compounding" was prominent in the reporting, putting all compounding activities in an unfavorable light. This horrible tragedy was caused by a calculation error *in one pharmacy in one location.* This situation gave all of compounding a black eye that was difficult to recover from. Even though it was "sterile" compounding, the public was not given information about the distinction between sterile and non-sterile, and compounding was the word that stuck in their minds. Nearly all public knowledge of compounding comes from these types of situations, and the view of compounding comes from the media. (Thomas K. Polo ponies were given incorrect medication. *New York Times.* April 23, 2009. http://www.nytimes.com/2009/04/24/sports/othersports/24polo.html?_r=0. Accessed August 28, 2014.)

1. Can you suggest some ways the compounding misconception be remedied?
2. Can you explain what the difference is between sterile and non-sterile compounding?
3. As a technician, what steps can you take to prevent calculation errors?

SCENARIO 2

You are covered by a group health plan (through the pharmacy where you are employed) with a formulary (lists of medications that they will pay for) that includes certain compounded prescription medications. These medications are often chosen because of their clinical efficacy and cost-effectiveness. One pharmacy filling these prescriptions is not located in the state where you live. The state board of pharmacy in your state discovers that this pharmacist is not licensed in your state and demands that the pharmacy discontinue selling the medication you need in your state.

Think of some options for yourself and others in this situation.

Answers to PTCB Review Questions

1. **C**
2. **C**
3. **D**
4. **A**
5. **D**
6. **D**
7. **A**
8. **C**
9. **D**
10. **A**

CHAPTER

2 Calculation Refresher

INTRODUCTION

Now that we have an understanding of what compounding entails, we need to master how to properly and accurately complete the calculations that are common in compounding practice. Accuracy is crucial, as one decimal point or a zero placed incorrectly can cause serious harm to a patient. All calculations should be double checked for precision, and *always* use a calculator to ensure that the math is done correctly. You may have already learned some of the concepts discussed in this chapter; the difference will be how it is used in the compounding of medications. As we continue through this text, there will be calculation problems at the end of each chapter to help reinforce the concepts introduced. When working as a pharmacy technician, if you are ever unsure of how to do a calculation or if you have questions regarding your answer, always ask the pharmacist.

LEARNING OBJECTIVES

- Define the metric system of measurement.
- Define the household system of measurement.
- Perform conversions between and within the metric and household measurement system.
- Understand the international/military time system.
- Perform conversions between the 24- and 12-hour time systems (international and traditional systems).
- Perform conversions between Celsius and Fahrenheit temperature systems.
- Understand and perform calculations using the alligation method.
- Understand and perform calculations using ratio/proportion.
- Understand and perform calculations using dimensional analysis.
- Understand regulation and laws pertaining to compounding.
- Understand and use non-sterile compounding resources.

Pharmacy technicians must be able to do accurate calculations in every situation in order to ensure the efficacy of the compounded products and the safety of the patient.

KEY TERMS

Alligation: A mathematical method used to add two different concentrations together to obtain a desired strength

Celsius (C): A system used to measure temperature outside the United States and in science or medicine

Denominator: The bottom of mathematical fractional expression that indicates the total of all parts

Dimensional analysis: A mathematical process that uses conversion factors to move from one unit of measurement to another

Fahrenheit (F): A system used to measure temperature, commonly used in the United States

Gram: A term used in the metric system to measure weight

Household system: System used in the United States to measure volume, length, and weight

Kilo: A prefix in the metric system that represents one thousand units

Liter: A term used in the metric system to measure volume

Meter: A term used in the metric system to measure length

Metric system: System used outside the United States and in science and medicine to measure volume, length, and weight

Micro: A prefix in the metric system representing one millionth

Military or universal time: A system used to measure time using a 24-hour clock

Milli: A prefix in the metric system representing one thousandth

Numerator: The top of a mathematical fractional expression that indicates parts of a whole

Ratio/proportion: A mathematical process used to solve equations showing an equal value

Solute: A substance that can be dissolved in another substance to create a solution

Solvent: A substance capable of dissolving another substance in order to create a solution

WEIGHT AND VOLUME CONVERSIONS

The household measurement "cup" should never be abbreviated as "C" because the pharmacy sig code "c" means "with" and the Roman numeral "C" is 100.

There are many systems that can be used to weigh and measure specific items. The most familiar system of measurement in the United States is the household system. This includes feet, inches, and yards for measuring length; ounces and pounds for weighing solids; and teaspoons, tablespoons, gallons, and pints for measuring and weighing liquids (Table 2-1).

In the world of medicine and science, the **metric system** is most commonly used to measure medications and substances. The metric system uses increments of 10 and prefixes to represent the units of measurement.

TABLE 2-1 Household Measurement System

Weight	Ounce (oz) Pound (lb)
Length	Feet (ft) Inches (in) Yards (yd)
Volume	Teaspoon (tsp) Tablespoon (tbsp) Cup Pint (pt) Quart (qt) Gallon (gal)

The Household System

A pharmacy technician must be able to convert between the household and metric system as well as within each system.

When we think of the **household system**, we often think of food. A recipe will call for specific amounts of ingredients that are combined together to create something to eat. Often, a physician will use these household terms when writing a prescription for the patient. Pharmacy technicians must be familiar with the terms and conversions within the household system. Measuring substances using this system is less accurate because the utensils used for measurement are not manufactured for scientific or medical use, and can sometimes vary greatly in size (Table 2-2).

The Metric System

The metric system is the measurement system used in the medical and pharmaceutical industry and in most countries outside the United States. It uses multiples of 10 so converting within the system is simple.

The metric system uses the following base measurements for liquid, weight, and length:

Liter: for measuring volume

Gram: for measuring weight

Meter: for measuring length (this is not commonly used in pharmacy calculations, so we will not discuss length in detail)

These usually have a prefix before them that represents a specific measurement. Common prefixes include:

Kilo: one thousand

Milli: one thousandth

Micro: one millionth

TABLE 2-2 Household Measurement Chart

Units (volume)	Conversion
1 tsp	
3 tsp	1 tbsp
2 tbsp	1 fl oz
8 fl oz	1 cup
2 cups	1 pt
2 pt	1 qt
4 qt	1 gal
Units (weight)	**Conversion**
1 lb	16 oz
Units (length)	**Conversion**
1 in	
1 ft	12 in
1 yard	3 ft
1 mile	1760 yards

fl oz, fluid ounce; ft, foot; gal, gallon; in, inch; lb, pound; oz, ounce; pt, pint; qt, quart; tbsp, tablespoonful; tsp, teaspoonful

For example, the prefix milli is placed before "gram" so the term "milligram" will represent a specific unit of measure.

There are a lot of prefixes that can measure both very large and very minute amounts. As a compounding technician, it is important to have a complete understanding of the most common prefixes used to measure substances in the pharmacy and in medical practice (Table 2-3).

TABLE 2-3 Common Metric System Prefixes and Terms Used in Pharmacy

Prefix/Term	Kilo-	Gram	Milli-	Micro-
Values	1 kilogram (kg) = 1000 grams (g)		1 gram = 1000 milligrams (mg)	1 milligram = 1000 micrograms (mcg)
Prefix/Term	**Kilo-**	**Liter**	**Mill-**	**Micro-**
Values	1 kiloliter (kL) = 1000 liters (L)		1 liter = 1000 milliliters (mL)	1 milliliter = 1000 microliters (mcL)

Some medications will be prescribed in g/L, while many others will be in mg/mL. It is important to be able to easily convert from one unit to another. An easy way of converting is moving the decimal point. When units are lined up from biggest to smallest, the decimal point is moved in the same direction and *three places* for each unit (Table 2-4).

TABLE 2-4 Biggest to Smallest Metric Units

Weight	Kilogram (kg)	Grams (g)	Milligram (mg)	Microgram (mcg)
Volume	Kiloliter (kL)	Liters (L)	Milliliter (mL)	Microliter (mcL)

EXAMPLE 1

2 mg = _______ g

0002 move the decimal point 3 places to the *left*

Answer: 2 mg = 0.002 g

EXAMPLE 2

0.002 g = ________mg

0.002 move the decimal point 3 places to the *right*

→

Answer: 0.002 g = 2 mg

EXAMPLE 3

If we were converting into kL, we would move the decimal point 6 places to the left because we are converting units twice.

20 mL = 0.02 L = 0.00002 kL

←

Moving the decimal point is a quick and easy way to obtain the unit required.

Converting Between the Household and Metric Systems

A prescription or medication order may be written by a physician using the household system, so it is imperative that a technician calculating a dosage or ingredients for a compounded product be able to convert from the household system to the metric system. Table 2-5 shows the conversions commonly used in the pharmacy.

TABLE 2-5 Household to Metric Conversions Used in Pharmacy

	Conversion
1 tsp	5 mL
1 tbsp	15 mL
1 fl oz	30 mL
1 cup	240 mL
1 pt	480 mL
1 qt	960 mL
1 gal	3840 mL
Household Unit	**Metric Conversion**
16 oz =1 lb	454 g
2.2 lb	1 kg
1 oz	28.4 g (often rounded to 30 g)

EXAMPLE 1

Suppose a baby weighs 6 lb and 4 oz, what is his weight kg?

Using Table 2-5, we know that 2.2 lb is equal to 1 kg.

So we divide

$$6.4 \text{ (lb)} \div 2.2 = 2.9 \text{ kg}$$

EXAMPLE 2

If a patient is prescribed 4 oz of magic mouthwash, how many milliliters are needed?

Using Table 2-5, we know that 1oz is equal 30 mL.

So we multiply

$$4 \times 30 = 120 \text{ mL}$$

There are several ways to do more complex conversion calculations; these are discussed in detail in the ratio/proportion and dimensional analysis section of this chapter.

TIME AND TEMPERATURE CONVERSIONS

Celsius and Fahrenheit

In addition to the importance of conversions for weight and volume, it is essential that a pharmacy technician be able to convert between the temperature systems **Fahrenheit (F)** and **Celsius (C)**. Pharmaceutical products and active ingredients used in compounding often need to be kept within specific temperature ranges to ensure their potency and stability. Fahrenheit (F) is the system that we are familiar with in the United States, but, like the metric system, Celsius (C) is the measurement system for temperature that is used in the medical world and outside the United States.

There are simple formulas that are used to convert between the two temperature systems (Table 2-6).

TABLE 2-6 Formulas for Converting Temperature

Fahrenheit (F°) to Celsius (C°)
F° − 32 ÷ 1.8 = C°
Celsius (C°) to Fahrenheit (F°)
C° × 1.8 + 32 = F°

To convert between the two systems, plug the appropriate numbers into the equation and complete the math.

EXAMPLE 1

F° − 32 ÷ 1.8 = C°

Step 1: Replace F° with our temperature (45).

45 − 32 = 13

Step 2: Divide the answer to the first equation by 1.8.

13 ÷ 1.8 = 7.2

Step 3: We have our completed our conversion problem.

45°F = 7.2°C

EXAMPLE 2

C° × 1.8 + 32 = F°

Step 1: Replace C° with our temperature (7.2, from example 1).

7.2 × 1.8 = 12.96

Step 2: Add 32 to the product.

12.96 + 32 = 44.96

Step 3: We have our completed our conversion problem.

7.2°C = 45°F

Time

Medical facilities document time in a system is known as **military or universal time**. This differs from the time system most Americans are familiar with. The military time system uses a 24-hour clock, whereas the US time system runs on a 12-hour clock and designates AM (before 12:00 noon) and PM (after 12:00 noon until midnight). In the military time system, the clock continues to move forward after 12:00 PM. Therefore, instead of the next hour reading as 1:00 PM, the military system reads 1300. Table 2-7 illustrates both these systems.

Notice that the military time system is written slightly differently. Besides not using the AM or PM designation, it also does not use a colon between the hour and minutes. For example, 5:15 AM would be written in military time as 0515, and 5:15 PM as 1715.

TABLE 2-7 The 12- and 24-hour Time Conversion Chart

12-h Clock	24-h Clock (Military or Universal Time System)
1:00 AM	0100 hours
2:00 AM	0200 hours
3:00 AM	0300 hours
4:00 AM	0400 hours
5:00 AM	0500 hours
6:00 AM	0600 hours
7:00 AM	0700 hours
8:00 AM	0800 hours
9:00 AM	0900 hours
10:00 AM	1000 hours
11:00 AM	1100 hours
12:00 noon	1200 hours
1:00 PM	1300 hours
2:00 PM	1400 hours
3:00 PM	1500 hours
4:00 PM	1600 hours
5:00 PM	1700 hours
6:00 PM	1800 hours
7:00 PM	1900 hours
8:00 PM	2000 hours
9:00 PM	2100 hours
10:00 PM	2200 hours
11:00 PM	2300 hours
12:00 Midnight	2400 hours (may also be written as 0000 hours)

EXAMPLE

1:30 PM is written 1330 in military time.
9:45 AM is written 0945 in military time.

ALLIGATIONS

Alligations are used frequently in non-sterile compounding to combine different strengths of separate active ingredients to create a new strength or a combination product. Accurately performing the alligation process is an imperative skill for all pharmacy personnel.

The alligation process uses a "tic-tac-toe"-type graph and a series of steps to perform an accurate calculation. We can use the acronym SAMD to help us remember the steps and their order:

Subtract
Add
Multiply
Divide

The easiest way to explain this process is to see an example.

EXAMPLE 1

A prescription calls for 40 g of hydrocortisone cream 12%. The pharmacy has 5% and 20% hydrocortisone formulations. How much of each strength will be needed to fill the prescription?

Step 1

Set up an alligation grid (tic-tac-toe).

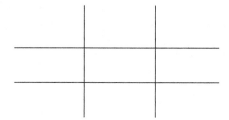

Step 2

Place the *final, desired* concentration in the center box of the grid (12%).

	12%	← Desired

Step 3

Place the high concentration in the upper-left corner of the grid (20%).

High 0% →		
	12%	

Step 4

Place the low concentration in the lower-left corner (5%).

20%		
	12%	
Low 5% →		

Step 5 (Subtract)

Subtract *diagonally* to determine the *number of parts needed* for each concentration. Subtract the low concentration from the concentration ordered.

$$12 - 5 = 7$$

Place the answer in the upper-right corner.

20		7 parts
	12	
5		

Step 6 (Subtract)

Subtract the concentration ordered from the high concentration.

$$20 - 12 = 8$$

Place the answer in the lower-right corner.

20		7
	12	
5		8 parts

Step 7 (Add)

Add the parts needed for each concentration to determine the *total number of parts* in the compound.

7 + 8 = 15 *total parts*

Step 8 (Multiply)

Multiply the number of parts of *each concentration* by the *total amount* ordered. (Remember from the prescription that the final amount is 40 g.)

20		$7 \times 40 = 280$
	12	
5		$8 \times 40 = 320$

Step 9 (Divide)

Divide each concentration by the total number of parts to determine the amount needed of each concentration. (Refer to step 7, total parts = 15.)

20		$7 \times 40 = 280$
	12	
5		$8 \times 40 = 320$

$$280 \div 15 = 18.7$$

$$320 \div 15 = 21.3$$

A script calls for 40 g of hydrocortisone cream 12%. Your pharmacy stocks both 5% and 20% formulations. How much of each strength will you need to fill this prescription?
Therefore, in order to correctly fill the prescription, we need

18.7 g of 20% hydrocortisone

21.3 g of 5% hydrocortisone

To easily check if your calculation was correct, add the amounts of both ingredients. The total should equal the total grams needed to fill the prescription.

$$18.7 + 21.3 = 40$$

40 g is the total needed so we did this correctly!

EXAMPLE 2

Coal tar gel 3.5% dispense 4 oz (120 g).
The pharmacy stocks coal tar 5% and clear gel base.
How much of each is needed to create the final product?

Step 1

Set up an alligation grid (tic-tac-toe).

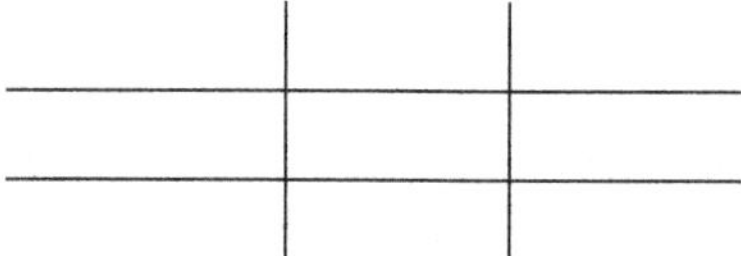

Step 2

Place the final, desired concentration in the center box of the grid.

	3.5%	

Step 3

Place the high concentration in the upper-left corner of the grid.

5%		
	3.5%	

Step 4

Place the low concentration in the lower-left corner.
In this case, the clear gel base is *not* an API so the percent strength is zero.

Any ingredient not considered and API (active pharmacy ingredient) will have a percent strength of zero.

2%		
	3.5%	
0%		

Step 5

Subtract *diagonally* to determine the *number of parts needed* for each concentration. Subtract the low concentration from the concentration ordered.

$$3.5 - 0 = 3.5$$

Place the answer in the upper-right corner.

5		3.5 parts
	3.5	
0		

Step 6

Subtract the concentration ordered from the high concentration.

$$5 - 3.5 = 1.5$$

Place the answer in the lower-right corner.

5		3.5
	3.5	
0		1.5 parts

Step 7

Add the parts needed for each concentration to determine the *total number of parts* in the compound.

$$3.5 + 1.5 = 5 \textit{ total parts}$$

Step 8

Multiply the number of parts of *each concentration* by the *total amount* ordered. (Remember from the prescription that the final amount is 120 g.)

5		3.5 × 120 = 420
	3.5	
0		1.5 × 120 = 180

Step 9

Divide each concentration by the total number of parts to determine the amount needed of each concentration. (Refer to step 7, total parts = 5.)

5		3.5 × 120 = 420
	3.5	
0		1.5 × 120 = 180

$$420 \div 5 = 84$$
$$180 \div 5 = 36$$

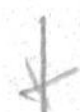

Coal tar gel 3.5% dispense 4 oz (120 g). The pharmacy stocks coal tar 5% and clear gel base. How much of each is needed to create the final product?

Therefore, in order to correctly fill the prescription we need

84 g of coal tar 5%

36 g of clear gel base

To easily check if your calculation was correct, add the amounts of both ingredients. The total should equal the total grams needed to fill the prescription.

$$84 + 36 = 120$$

120 g is the total amount prescribed. So our calculations are correct!

RATIO/PROPORTION AND DIMENSIONAL ANALYSIS

Many calculations for compounding can be done using one of two methods: **Ratio/proportion** is useful when we know 3 of the 4 values. The missing value can be calculated by understanding that a proportion is an *equality* of two **ratios**. Another method of obtaining drug dosages is **dimensional analysis.** This method utilizes the canceling of units so that the unit that remains in the **numerator** *is* the one for which we are solving. An example of each will make it easier to understand how both these calculations are done.

Ratio/Proportion

EXAMPLE 1 (Ratio/Proportion)

If we are dispensing 150 mL bottle of medication and the dose is 12.5 mL, how many doses does this quantity contain?

Step 1: To determine the dosage, set up 2 equal ratios.

Step 2: Make your unknown (X) the number of *doses*.

Make sure to keep all units on the top the same and all units on the bottom the same.

$$\frac{X \text{ (number of doses)}}{150 \text{ mL}} = \frac{1 \text{ dose}}{12.5 \text{ mL}}$$

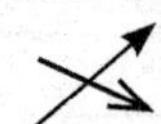

(*Continued on next page*)

Step 3: Now cross multiply and divide.

$$150 \times 1 = 150$$
$$150 \div 12.5 = 12$$
$$X = 12$$

Therefore this bottle contains 12 doses of 12.5 mL.

When calculating dosages using ratio/proportion, it is important to remember that the values in the *numerators must be the same unit*, and the numbers in the denominators *must also be the same units*.

Don't forget to *round* your answer if necessary.

EXAMPLE 2 (Ratio/Proportion)

If a patient is to receive 14 mg of oral diphenhydramine liquid and it is only available as 5 mg/mL, how many milliliters are needed for each dose?

Step 1: Set up two equal ratios.

Step 2: Make your unknown (X) the *mL needed per dose.*

$$\frac{\text{X mL per dose}}{\text{14 mg}} = \frac{\text{1 mL}}{\text{5 mg}}$$

Step 3: Cross multiply and divide.

$$\frac{\text{X mL}}{\text{14 mg}} = \frac{\text{1 mL}}{\text{5 mg}}$$

$$14 \times 1 = 14$$
$$14 \div 5 = 2.8$$
$$X = 2.8$$

That means our patient will need to receive 2.8 mL of diphenhydramine 5 mg/mL oral liquid for every dose.

Dimensional Analysis

EXAMPLE 1 (Dimensional Analysis)

If a patient is to receive 14 mg of diphenhydramine oral liquid and it is only available as 5 mg/mL, how many milliliters will be needed per dose?

Step 1: The *dose* is our *numerator* 14 mg.

Step 2: Multiply this by the *ratio* of medication: 5 mg/mL (5 mg:1 mL).

$$\text{14 mg} \times \frac{\text{1 mL}}{\text{5 mg}}$$

mg is both the numerator and denominator

Step 3: Cancel units (both the *units* in the numerator and denominator should be the same, so they can be cancelled).

$$14\ \cancel{\text{mg}} \times \frac{\text{1 mL}}{5\ \cancel{\text{mg}}}$$

Remember we are solving for milliliter (this is the units we have left).

Step 4: *Multiply* all values in the numerators and then *divide* by all values in the denominator.

$$14 \times 1 = 14 \div 5 = 2.8 \text{ mL}$$

Therefore the patient will receive 2.8 mL of oral diphenhydramine 5 mg/mL for each dose.

When using *dimensional analysis*, the *units* in the *numerator* and *denominator* must be the *same* so they can be cancelled.

Either ratio/proportion or dimensional analysis can also be used to calculate doses based on weight. Weight-based dosing is important in pediatric and geriatric populations.

If a weight is given in pounds, Always convert pounds to kilograms.(1 kg = 2.2 lb)

EXAMPLE 2 (Dimensional Analysis: Weight-Based Dosing)

A patient weighs 128 lb and is to receive a medication of 4 mg/kg. What is this patient's dose?

Step 1: Convert pounds to kilograms.

$$128 \div 2.2 = 58.18 \text{ kg (round to 58.2 kg)}$$

Step 2: The patient's weight is our *numerator*.

$$\frac{58.2 \text{ kg}}{} \times \frac{4 \text{ mg}}{1 \text{ kg}}$$

Step 3: Cancel *like* units.

$$\frac{58.2 \cancel{\text{kg}}}{} \times \frac{4 \text{ mg}}{1 \cancel{\text{kg}}}$$

Step 4: Multiply the numerators and divide by the denominator.

$$58.2 \times 4 = 232.8 \div 1 = 232.8$$

The patient will need to receive 232.8 mg.

Step 5: Round the dose (this is true in *most* cases, but some dosing will need to be exact; check with the pharmacist to make sure it is okay to round).

232.8 mg *rounded* is 233 mg.

PERCENT AND RATIO STRENGTH (W/V, W/W, V/V)

Compounding technicians will often encounter medications that require further dilution to create a new desired strength.

A substance (ie, powder) that is *dissolved* in a liquid is known as the **solute**. The liquid itself is known as the **solvent**. This is discussed in more detail in upcoming chapters of this text.

A solution that contains a greater amount of solute is considered to be more concentrated than a solution containing more solvent. For example, if you added 30 g of salt to 1 gal of water and 30 g of salt to a ½ gal of water, the ½ gal of solution would be more *concentrated* because there will be more *solute (salt)* per milliliters of solvent. The *percent strength* represents how much active ingredient is in 100 mL or 100 g of a final product.

This is an important concept expressed in 3 types of ratios:

w/v (weight in volume) = is number of *grams* of active ingredient per *100 mL* of total solution.

w/w (weight in weight) = number of *grams* of active ingredient per *100 g* of total product.

v/v (volume in volume) = number of *milliliters* of active ingredient in *100 mL* of total solution.

For example, a 12% solution or powder is expressed as the following:

The percent strength represents how much active ingredient is in 100 mL or 100 g of a final product.

When determining the percent strength, the ratio is always multiplied by 100.

w/v = 12 g/100 mL = 12% (12 g of active ingredient in 100 mL)

w/w = 12 g/100 g = 12% (12 g of active ingredient in 100 g)

v/v =12 mL/100 mL = 12% (12 mL of active ingredient in 100 mL)

When the percent strength of a product is known, we can then determine how much active ingredient is in a specified amount of medication using either ratio/proportion or dimensional analysis.

EXAMPLE 1: (Ratio/Proportion)

How many grams of zinc oxide are in 80 g of a 12% ointment?

Step 1: Write the percent strength as a w/w ratio or fraction.

$$12\% = \frac{12}{100}$$

(Continued on next page)

Step 2: Make your unknown (X) the amount of zinc oxide needed.

$$\frac{X}{80} = \frac{12}{100}$$

Step 3: Cross multiply and divide.

$$12 \times 80 = 960$$

$$960 \div 100 = 9.6$$

In order to produce 80 g of 12% ointment, we will need 9.6 g of zinc oxide.

EXAMPLE 2: (Dimensional Analysis)

How much hydrogen peroxide is contained in 450 mL of 3% hydrogen peroxide solution?

Step 1: Write the percent strength in a v/v ratio or fraction.

$$3\% = \frac{3}{100}$$

Step 2: Set up your equation using your final volume as the numerator.

$$\frac{450\text{ mL}}{} = \frac{3\text{ mL}}{100\text{ mL}}$$

Step 3: Cancel like units (since this is v/v equation, all the units are alike).

$$\frac{450\ \cancel{\text{mL}}}{} = \frac{3\text{ mL}}{100\ \cancel{\text{mL}}}$$

Step 4: Multiply the numerators, divide by the denominator.

$$450 \times 3 = 1350 \div 100 = 13.5$$

There are 13.5 mL of hydrogen peroxide in 450 mL of the 3% solution.

Let's do one more using both calculation methods.

How many grams of lidocaine are needed to prepare 150 mL of 2% lidocaine solution?

Ratio/Proportion

Step 1: Write the percent strength as a ratio or fraction.

$$2\% = \frac{2}{100}$$

Step 2: Set up your equation.

$$\frac{X}{150} = \frac{2}{100}$$

Step 3: Cross multiply to solve for X.

$$2 \times 150 = 300$$

$$300 \div 100 = 3$$

Dimensional Analysis

How many grams of lidocaine are needed to prepare 150 mL of 2% lidocaine solution?

Step 1: Write the percent strength as a ratio or fraction.

$$2\% = \frac{2}{100}$$

Step 2: Set up your equation, using the final volume as your numerator.

$$\frac{150\text{ mL}}{} = \frac{2\text{ grams}}{100\text{ mL}}$$

(Continued on next page)

Step 3: Cancel like units.

$$= \frac{150 \cancel{\text{mL}} \times \frac{2 \text{ grams}}{}}{100 \cancel{\text{mL}}}$$

Step 4: Multiply the numerators, divide by the denominator.

$$150 \times 2 = 300 \div 100 = 3$$

Using either method, we come up with the same answer; to prepare our 150 mL of our 2% solution, we will need 3 g of lidocaine. Great Job!

CONCLUSION

Pharmacy technicians perform many different calculations in *every* practice setting, so it is important that you are comfortable completing the different types of problems discussed in this chapter. *Remember to always double-check your calculation and use a calculator when doing any medical math, as this could potentially cause harm to the patient.* The key to learning calculations is repetition, so if you are still having trouble with any of the equations or methods described in this chapter, ask the pharmacist, your instructor, or use the Internet or a math textbook to get some additional practice.

CHAPTER SUMMARY

- Always use a calculator when doing medical math, and double-check your work.
- Measuring volumes using household measurement is less accurate because of the variety in size of measuring utensils.
- When converting within the metric system from a unit that is larger into a smaller unit (eg, kL to L), the decimal point should be moved to the right.
- When converting within the metric system from a unit that is smaller into a larger unit (eg, mcL to mL), the decimal point should be moved to the left.
- The decimal point is moved in the same direction and 3 places for each unit within the decimal system.
- Military time (also known as *international time*) is used in most medical settings.
- Military time operates on a 24-hour clock. AM and PM are not necessary.
- Drug stability and potency are often based on specific temperature and storage requirements.
- An alligation should be used to add 2 different concentrations together to obtain a desired strength.
- Ratio/proportion and dimensional analysis are the common ways for pharmacy calculation equations.
- The units in the numerator must match, and units in the denominator must match in a ratio/proportion equation.
- The same units should be in the numerator and denominator so they can be cancelled when solving problems using dimensional analysis.
- Weight-based dosing is often used for calculating geriatric and pediatric doses.
- 1 kg is equal to 2.2 lb.
- Weight calculations are provided as milligrams of a medication per kilogram of body weight.
- To determine percentage strength, a ratio is multiplied by 100.

PTCB Review Questions

1. If a patient receives 2 tsp at bedtime of diphenhydramine oral solution 5 mg/5 mL, what are the total milliliters needed for a 7-day regimen?
   A. 77 mL
   B. 35 mL
   C. 70 mL
   D. 350 mL
2. Convert 78.4°C (Celsius) to Fahrenheit (F).
   A. 173.1°F
   B. 141°F
   C. 156.8°F
   D. 12°F
3. A patient needs to take his medication every day at 2 PM. If he/she is admitted to the hospital, how is that documented on his/her inpatient medication order?
   A. 2:00 PM
   B. 2200 hours
   C. 0200 hours
   D. 1400 hours
4. What are the steps in order of operation needed to solve an alligation equation?
   A. Add, subtract, divide, multiply
   B. Subtract, multiply, divide
   C. Subtract, add, multiply, divide
   D. Cross multiply and divide
5. If a patient weighing 134 lb is prescribed 3 mg/kg of an oral medication, how many milligrams of medication are needed per dose?
   A. 61 mg
   B. 183 mg
   C. 402 mg
   D. None of the above
6. A prescription is written for 90 g of a 5% topical ointment. It is only available in a 1.5% and 4% concentration. How many grams of each available concentration will be needed to fill the prescription?
   A. 70 g of 1.5% and 20 g of 4%
   B. 20 g of 1.5% and 70 g of 4%
   C. 50 g of 4% and 40 g of 1.5%
   D. 10 g of 1.5% and 80 g of 4%
7. If there are 12 g of medication in 250 mL of solution, what is the percent strength?
   A. 7.2%
   B. 72%
   C. 48%
   D. 4.8%
8. A patient weighs 135 lb. If a medication is to be given as 2 mg/kg twice daily for 5 days and the medication is available as 10 mg/mL, how many milliliters should be dispensed to the patient?
   A. 123 mL
   B. 130 mL
   C. 50 mL
   D. 61.4 mL
9. In what patient population is weight-based dosing often used?
   A. Pediatric
   B. Geriatric
   C. No patient populations ever use weight-based dosing
   D. Both A and B
10. Convert 88°F to Celsius
    A. 190°C
    B. 31.1°C
    C. 16.9°C
    D. 1.69°C

Techs in Practice: Discussion Topics and Questions

SCENARIO 1

You are asked to combine an API and a water-washable base to prepare 450 g of a 4% cream that is not commercially available. What kind of calculation is needed to come up with the desired product?

SCENARIO 2

Using the Internet or other resources, list common non-sterile compounding APIs that require refrigeration.

What is the range for storing APIs in the refrigerator?
List the temperature range in both Fahrenheit and Celsius.
What is the range for storing APIs at controlled room temperature?
List the temperature range in both Celsius and Fahrenheit.

Calculation Review Questions

1. The ingredients for a compounded lollipop must be heated to 155°C. The thermometer in the pharmacy reads only Fahrenheit. Convert 155°C to Fahrenheit in order to follow the directions in the formulation.
2. Each day, the temperature of the refrigerator in the compounding area must be logged. The centigrade thermometer in the refrigerator is broken and only the Fahrenheit thermometer is available. Convert the following daily temperature readings to Fahrenheit.

   3.4°C
   6.7°C
   5°C

3. A prescription is to dispense 30 g of nifedipine 0.2% ointment. The instruction is to use a commercially available 2% nifedipine ointment and white petrolatum to prepare this medication. Using alligation, calculate the proper amount of nifedipine ointment and white petrolatum needed to fill the prescription.
4. A dermatologist has prescribed a 50% glycolic acid solution for a patient. Glycolic acid is supplied as a 70% solution in water. Write the alligation needed to calculate how much glycolic acid 70% solution and how much water will be required to prepare 100 mL of the 50% glycolic acid solution needed to fill the prescription.
5. The physician has ordered a compounded oseltamivir (Tamiflu) suspension to be shared by 3 pediatric patients in 1 family. Tamiflu is dosed by weight. The suspension is to be prepared from Tamiflu capsules in a concentration of 15 mg/mL. Calculate the amount of the suspension which will be administered to each of the 3 children *per dose* using the following information:

Weight (kg)	Dose (mg)
< 15	30
16-23	45
24-40	60
≥ 41	75

   Amy weighs 24 lb
   Craig weighs 40 lb
   Peter weighs 71 lb

6. A medication needs to be administered every 6 hours around the clock. The first dose is due at 8 AM each morning. Write a 24-hour dosing schedule in military/international time.
7. How many grams of hydrocortisone are in 45 g of a 30% cream?
8. The concentration of carvedilol compounded pediatric oral suspension is 1.67 mg/mL.

   How many mL are needed for a 4.5mg dose?
   If the patient receives 2 doses daily for 7 days, what is the total volume to be dispensed?

This chapter includes the following PTCE Blueprint Knowledge Areas

Section 1.0-1.4 Strengths/dose, dosage forms, physical appearance, routes of administration, and duration of drug therapy.

Section 3.0-3.7 Non-sterile compounding processes.

Section 4.0-4.3 Identify issues that require pharmacist intervention (eg, DUR, ADE, OTC recommendation, therapeutic substitution, misuse, missed dose).

Section 6.0-6.3 Calculate dose required.

Section 7.0-7.4 Storage requirements (eg, refrigeration, freezer, warmer).

This chapter includes the following Ex-CPT Test Specifications

Section 3 B-6 Follow the pharmacy's quality assurance policies and procedures.

Section 3 B-7 Follow proper procedures to avoid medication errors.

Section 3 C-1 Convert within and between each of the systems of measurement.

Section 3 C-2 Calculate the quantities of prescription medication to be dispensed.

Section 3 C-4 Properly calculate individual and daily dosages.

Section 3 C-5 Correctly perform compounding calculations (eg, ratio strength, w/w%, w/v%, v/v%, dilution/concentration, mEq)

Section 3 D-9 Compound and label sterile products accurately.

This chapter includes the following ASHP Model Curriculum for Pharmacy Technician Training Goal Statements, Objectives, and Instructional Objectives

OBJ 3.5 Accurately count or measure finished dosage forms as specified by the prescription/medication order.

OBJ 3.7 Accurately determine the correct amounts of ingredients for a compounded product.

OBJ 3.11 Follow safety policies and procedures in the preparation of all medications.

OBJ 15.1 Explain the characteristics of an effective pharmacy department approach to preventing medication misadventures.

OBJ 17.1 Act ethically in the conduct of all job-related activities.

Answers to PTCB Review Questions

1. **C**
2. **A**
3. **D**
4. **C**
5. **B**
6. **B**
7. **D**
8. **A**
9. **D**
10. **B**

Answers to Calculation Review Questions

1. 311°F
2. 38.1°F
   44°F
   41°F
3. 15.8 g of 2% nifedipine
   14.2 g of white petroleum
4. 71.4 mL of 70% glycolic acid
   28.6 mL of water
5. Amy 2 mL
   Craig 3 mL
   Peter 4 mL
6. 0800
   1400
   2000
   0200
7. 13.5 g hydrocortisone
8. 2.7 mL
   37.8 mL

CHAPTER 3

Tools, Supplies, and Equipment

INTRODUCTION

As you become more familiar with non-sterile compounding practices in various pharmacies, you will see many differences in the space and personnel dedicated to these compounding activities. Some pharmacies will have a small area, maybe just 6 to 8 ft of counter top with minor storage capacity and few pieces of equipment. Others will have larger operations, designed to prepare a significant number of compounded medications. Some pharmacies are **closed-door pharmacies** where compounding is the only activity performed. Most hospitals and health centers have areas devoted to non-sterile compounding as well. Whether the pharmacy has a full laboratory or a simple compounding area, you will see specific tools used in the preparation of prescription medications. This chapter familiarizes you with many of these items and some of the processes used in non-sterile compounding.

LEARNING OBJECTIVES

- Describe and explain the importance of equipment used to prepare non-sterile compounds.
- Describe the different types of balances used in pharmacy compounding.
- Describe the supplies needed to properly weigh materials used to compound medications.
- Explain balance certification and calibration.
- Explain cleaning procedures and personal protection equipment (PPE).
- Describe the different types of utensils and glassware used in a compounding environment.
- Explain the difference between "to make" and "to measure" as it pertains to compounding.
- Describe the different types of specialized equipment used in non-sterile compounding.
- Explain the purpose and importance of inventory management and equipment maintenance.

KEY TERMS

Analytical balance: An electronic balance used to measure weight that displays 4 places to the right of the decimal point; can accurately measure smaller quantities than a scientific balance

API: Active pharmaceutical ingredient

Balance: A precision instrument used to weigh substances

Beaker: A cylindrical container used for stirring, mixing, and heating liquids; most have a small spout for pouring and a flat bottom

Calibration weight: A weight used to verify that balance is working properly

Capacity: The highest amount that a balance can accurately measure

Cavity: A hollow area or hole that can be filled

Class A balance: A precision device used to measure pharmacy ingredients by weight; also known as a *torsion balance*

Closed-door pharmacy: A pharmacy that is not open to the public. It usually provides prescription drugs to nursing homes, long-term care facilities, and other institutional sites

Conical cylinder: A cone-shaped (wider at the top than at the bottom) device used to measure the volume of a liquid

Cross contamination: Unintentional transfer from one substance or object to another, which may result in a harmful effect

Draft shields: A device that keeps air movement from disturbing the accuracy of the balance

Electronic mortar and pestle (EMP): A device equipped with a powerful motor and settings for mixing speed and time; used to create a homogeneous mixture and uses specialized jars that can also be used for dispensing

Elliptical: Oval shaped

Final volume: The determined total amount of a liquid preparation

Formulation: Active drug and other substances combined together to create a specific dosage form

Glassine: A waxy substance applied to weigh papers; it keeps powder from sticking to it

Graduated cylinder: A straight sided device used to measure the volume of a liquid

Gross mixture: The first, rough combination of numerous ingredients

Homogeneous: Completely and evenly mixed

Mold: A frame or hollow cavity that determines the capacity and shape of a solid dosage form

Mortar and pestle (M&P): A mortar is a bowl, typically made of glass or ceramic. A pestle is a club-shaped object, in which the larger end is used for crushing or grinding.

MRL: Minimum reorder level

Ointment mill: A device that moves a cream or ointment through a set of ceramic rollers to create a homogeneous mixture

Ointment slab: A glass surface used to prepare ointments or creams

Lollipop: A lozenge or troche on a stick; often used for medication administration in children

Personal protection equipment (PPE): Garments and supplies used to protect compounded products from contaminants; provides a barrier between compounding personnel and the effects of substances used in a compounded preparation

Powder hood: A cabinet that pulls air away from the operator, carrying compounding powders into a set of high-efficiency particulate air (HEPA) filters; used to protect patients and staff from API powder residue

Rapid dissolve tablets (RDT): A dosage form that is placed on top of the tongue that dissolves quickly

Readability: The lowest amount that a balance can accurately measure

Scientific balance: An electronic balance used to measure weight that displays three places to the right of the decimal point; the most common type of balance used in a compounding pharmacy

Spatula: A flat-ended utensil used for mixing

Spatulation: The combining of materials by continuously heaping them together and smoothing them out using a spatula

Sublingual: A pharmacologic route of administration by which medication is diffused into the blood through tissues under the tongue

Suppository: A solid dosage form that is inserted into the rectum, vagina, or urethra

Tablet press: A mechanical device used in manufacturing that compresses powder into tablets of uniform size and weight

Tablet triturates (TT): A solid dosage form that quickly dissolves under the tongue

To make: A scale that indicates general measurements, used to indicate volume

To measure: A scale that indicates accurate measurements, used to indicate weight

Torsion balance: A 2-pan balance that utilizes both internal and external weights for precise measurement of ingredients used to compound pharmaceuticals

Triturate: To reduce particle size by rubbing or grinding

Troches (Lozenge): A solid dosage form that slowly dissolves in the buccal cavity (cheek)

Weigh boats or canoes: A disposable container used to hold powders as they are being weighed on a balance; used for larger quantities than can be contained on weighing papers

Weighing papers: A disposable paper used to contain powders on a balance

Vehicle: An inert medium to which an API is mixed or added

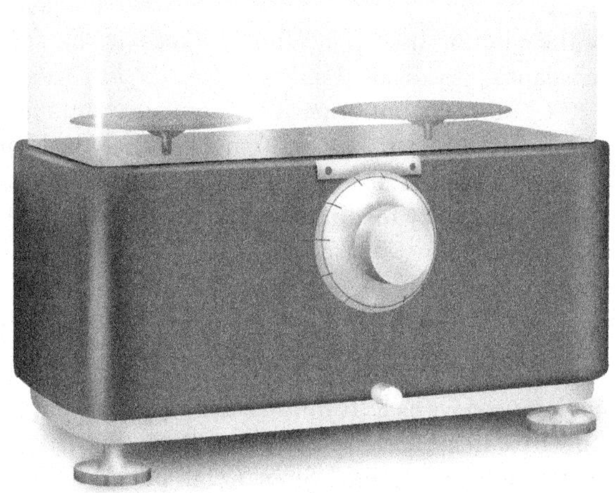

FIGURE 3-1 Torsion balance.

BALANCES

One of the most basic and necessary tools needed in compounding is a **balance**. A balance is a precision device that is used to measure ingredients by weight. A pharmacy of any kind must have a working **class A balance**, and the most basic of these is a **torsion balance** (Figure 3-1). A torsion balance has 2 pans that are attached to opposite ends of a lever and fulcrum. One end holds a calibrated weight and the other holds a pan to contain the ingredient being measured. To use a torsion balance in order to measure 5 g of a powder, a 5 g weight is placed on the base pan and powder is added to the weighing pan until the balance is level. While there are many torsion balances still in service, in a practice that compounds regularly, an electronic balance is now the modern standard of practice.

Electronic Balance

An electronic balance has just 1 pan, and instead of using an external weight to establish the target weight of the material being measured, it "reads" the weight of the material and displays the measurement on a light-emitting diode (LED) display (Figure 3-2). A **calibration weight** is used to verify that the balance is working properly. Validating this calibration is an important part of required compounding practices (Figure 3-3). Electronic balances have various capabilities and capacities representing the range of weights that can be accurately measured.

Balances are selected on the basis of two specifications: the greatest amount they can weigh accurately (**capacity**) and the least amount they can accurately weigh (**readability**). There are two types of balances used in a compounding pharmacy, a **scientific balance** and

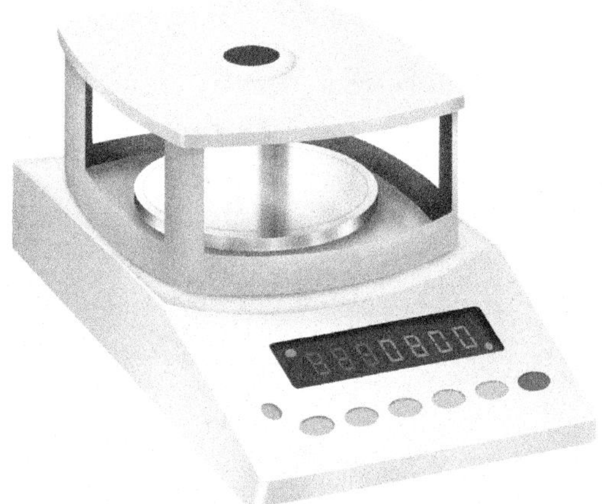

FIGURE 3-2 Electronic scientific balance.

an **analytical balance**. Either type of balance can have a *maximum* weigh capacity of 320 or 210 g accurate to *20%* of the amount displayed. While the capacity may vary, you will know you are using a scientific balance if the display shows *3 places to the right of the decimal point.* Because the accuracy is 20% of the amount displayed, the smallest amount that can be **accurately** weighed on a scientific balance is 0.02 g or 20 mg. An analytical balance has *4 places to the right of the decimal point*, and its readability is 20% of the smallest amount displayed or 0.002 g (2 mg). Because most pharmacy **formulations** that are compounded do not require an accurate measure of less than 20 mg, the scientific balance is the most common balance used in compounding (Table 3-1).

Supplies Used with Electronic Balances

There are a variety of supplies used with electronic balances. Weigh papers, boats, and canoes are common (Table 3-2). These items are disposable and lightweight, and are placed on the balance pan to hold the material being weighed. Some **weigh papers** are coated with **glassine**, a type of waxy material that releases the powders easily. **Weigh boats** are made of thin, flexible plastic and are square, round, or hexagon shaped. **Weigh canoes** are usually made of thicker material and have a spout on one side. Papers usually are used to weigh small amounts,while canoes and boats are used to weigh larger amounts of compounding ingredients (see Table 3-2). Spoons are used to remove powders from their bulk containers to be placed on a balance for proper measurement. A common type of spoon used is made of stainless steel, with an elliptical spoon on one end and a flat surface on the opposite end. The spoon end can retrieve large portions of powder, and the flat end allows easy removal of small amounts of material. Because many preparations require use of a tool to remove powders from containers, special attention must be paid to cleaning them. To prevent **cross contamination**, disposable spoons are becoming the trend, replacing stainless steel instruments that must be washed (see Table 3-2).

Draft Shield

Electronic balances are extremely sensitive to air movement. A **draft shield** is included with most electronic balances (see Figure 3-3). This accessory prevents air movement from disturbing the accuracy of the balance. A draft shield surrounds the pan and has a top. Some are tall and square, with doors on the sides that may be either hinged or slide open. It may be necessary

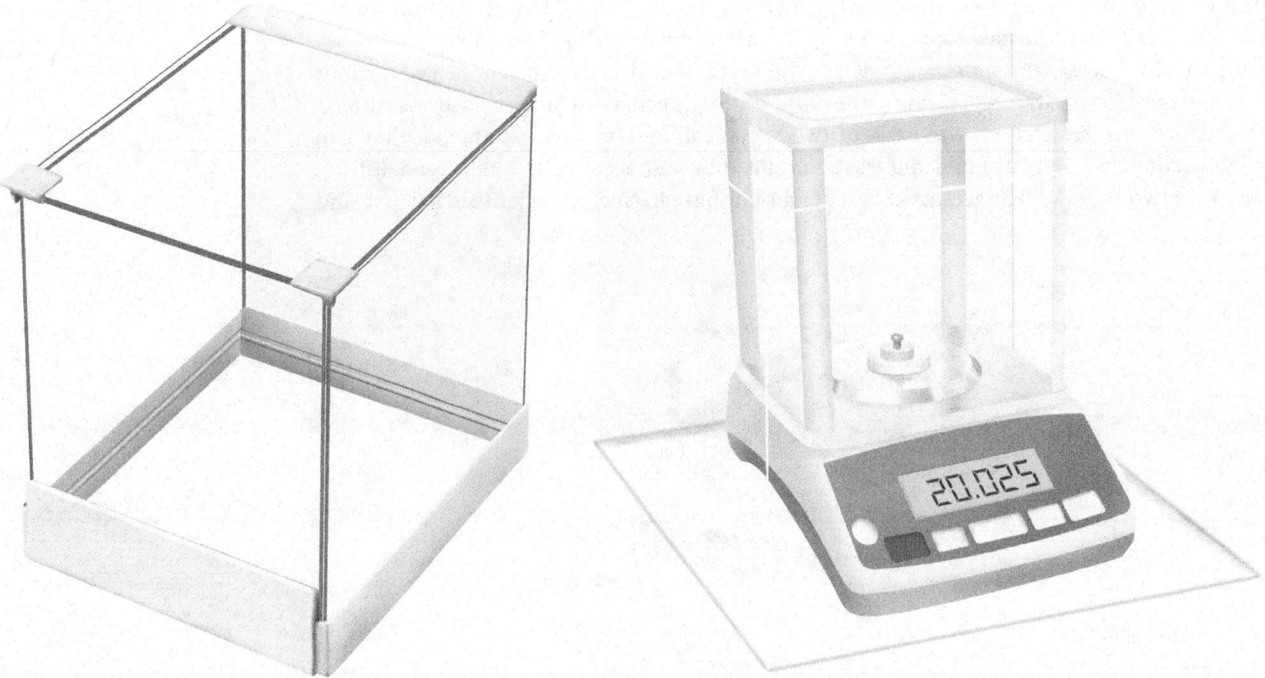

FIGURE 3-3 Draft shields.

TABLE 3-1 Scientific Balance Versus Analytical Balance

Scientific balance	Maximum weigh capacity: 320 or 210 g (depends on the balance) (see manufacture guide)	Accurate to 20 mg	3 places to the right of decimal point
Analytical balance	Maximum weigh capacity: 320 or 210 g (depends on the balance) (see manufacture guide)	Accurate to 2 mg	4 places to the right of decimal point

TABLE 3-2 Balance Supplies

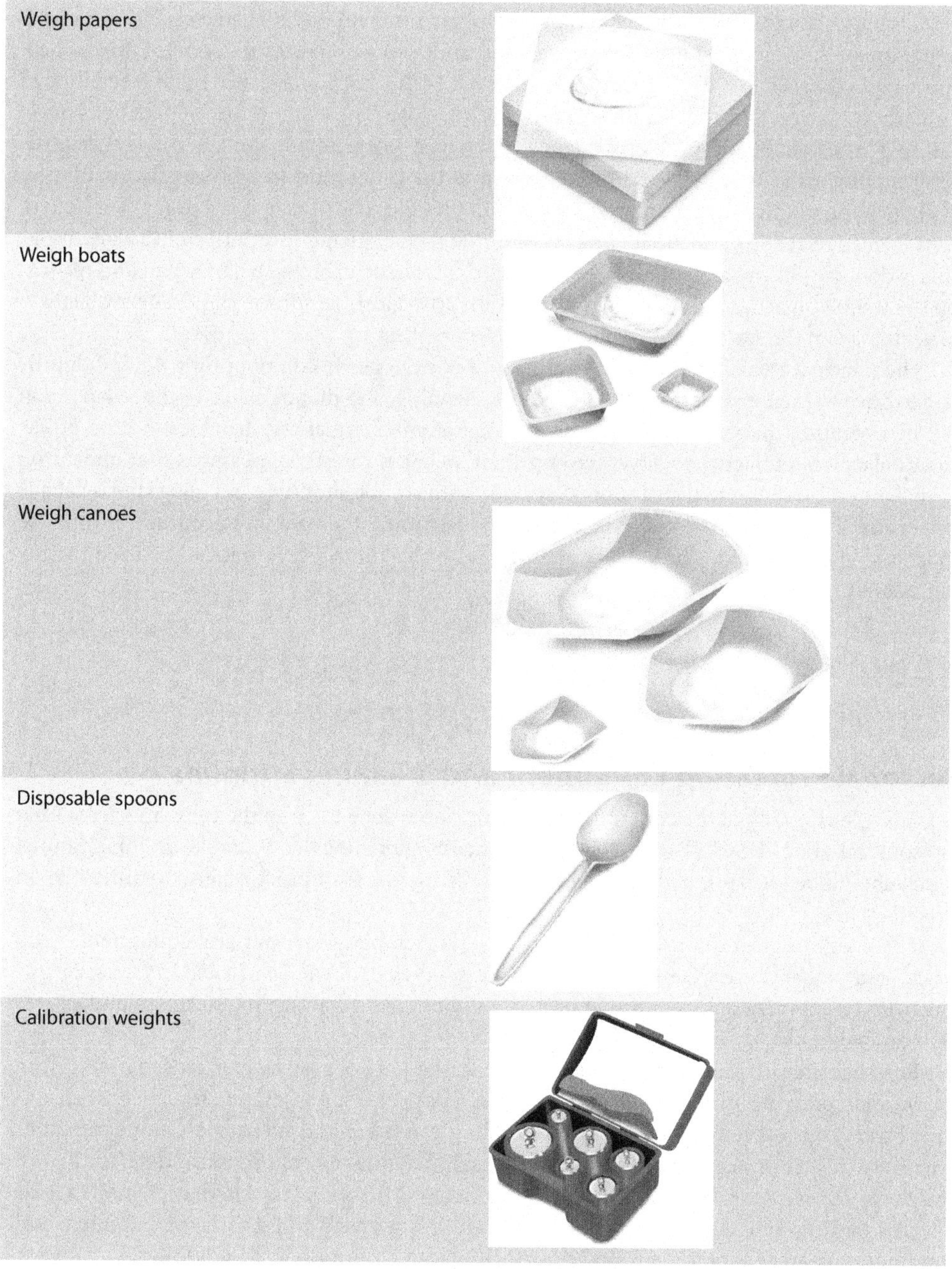

Weigh papers
Weigh boats
Weigh canoes
Disposable spoons
Calibration weights

to open the door and place the powder on the pan, and then close it to block air movement while the balance settles into the accurate reading. There are simple strategies for efficient manipulations of the draft shield. For example, if 5 g of powder is needed, leave the shield open until the display reads 4.900. Then close the door with each addition of small amounts of powder until the balance stabilizes at 5.000 g with the door closed.

Calibration and Documentation

Electronic balances are very delicate pieces of equipment. The first step in proper use of the electronic balance is to level it on the counter. Every balance has a level built into the base. The balance has at least two adjustable legs, usually the front feet, and these are adjusted to raise and/or lower opposing feet until a bubble inside the level is centered within a circular target.

It is important to note that there are specific instructions in USP/NF Chapter ⟨795⟩ for documentation of the accuracy of the balance. This includes securing recertification of the **calibration weight** (see Table 3-2) that is usually required each year. The balance must be calibrated regularly to ensure that the weight displayed is accurate. The calibration weight is normally sent to a local weight and measures agency of the local government similar to one that certifies gas pumps and truck scales. Recertification of the calibration weight usually qualifies as recertification of the balance, and the agency will provide a certificate of accuracy. Very often, technicians are required to perform calibration and documentation duties on a daily basis. This is done by placing a certified weight, usually 100 or 200 g, on the balance pan and recording the weight on a log. This daily log, as well the certificate of accuracy, should be available to inspectors from the state board of pharmacy upon request.

The pharmacy balance is an invaluable piece of non-sterile compounding equipment. Be sure to have written instructions on proper use, cleaning, and maintenance of the balance you will be operating. Become familiar with the operations manual and troubleshooting guide. Most balance manufacturers have help on their websites for error messages that appear on the balance display. Some distributors can assist with troubleshooting and have staff available for service if needed. If there is ever a question regarding the balance's accuracy, it must be addressed and corrected. The balance must then be recalibrated before it can be used for any compounding activities.

BASIC EQUIPMENT AND SUPPLIES USED FOR NON-STERILE COMPOUNDING

Personal Protection Equipment and Cleaning Supplies

A main responsibility of the compounding technician will be to clean the tools and areas used for compounding. USP/NF Chapter ⟨795⟩ contains guidelines and standards for cleaning, which should be incorporated into the pharmacy's standards of practice and documented on a regular basis.

There will be cleaning procedures and schedules in place for specialty equipment, work space, and reusable compounding utensils. *All equipment should be cleaned after each use.* Electronic equipment and removable parts should be cleaned according to the manufacture's recommendations.

Reusable utensils and equipment should be washed in hot soapy water, rinsed in hot clean water, and sprayed with 70% isopropyl alcohol (IPA). An automatic dishwasher is acceptable; however, spots left behind on compounding glassware and utensils are not acceptable. Therefore, if a dishwasher is used, an industrial machine and appropriate detergent must be selected to ensure complete cleaning and rinsing. Microfiber towels that do not include solvents or antiseptic are also acceptable for reusable utensils and glassware. Counters and compounding areas should be wiped down with clean cloth towels, disposable paper towels, or premoistened wipes approved for pharmacy use. Many compounding sites use disposable tools and supplies to avoid the risk of microbial bacteria growth and cross contamination between products.

Compounding personnel should wear clean scrubs or a lab coat. Other **personal protection equipment (PPE)** such as gloves, masks, paper gowns, and hair covers may also be

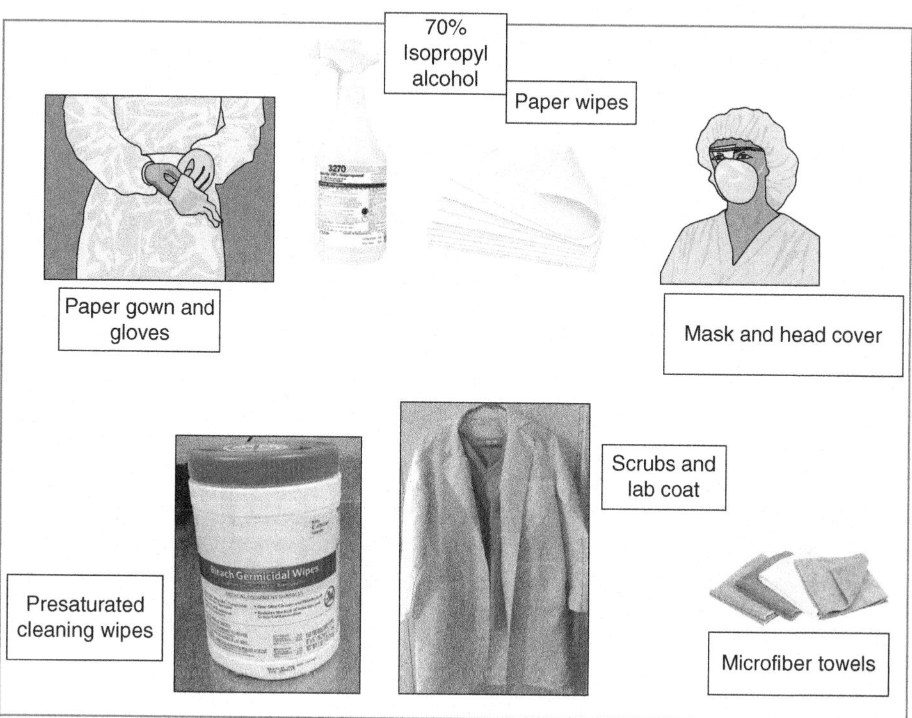

FIGURE 3-4 Examples of personal protection equipment and cleaning supplies.

required (Figure 3-4). PPE not only protects the compounded product from contaminants, but it also provides a barrier between compounding personnel and the effects of substances used in compounding. Hands should be washed thoroughly and often; nails should be kept trimmed and use of fragrance enhanced products should be avoided in a compounding area.

All compounding equipment and areas should be thoroughly cleaned after each use to avoid cross contamination and inhibit bacteria growth.

Glassware

In order to perform accurate pharmaceutical compounding, the pharmacists and technicians working in the compounding area will utilize various types of glassware for measuring and mixing compounded medications. Beakers and graduates are used to measure liquids. Pharmacy glassware items have measurement markings etched or printed on the exterior surface. These markings are classified as **to make** and **to measure**. "To make" markings are normally in increments of 5 or 10 mL. They are less accurate than "to measure" markings that usually appear in increments of 1 or 2 mL. Glassware with "to make" markings are commonly used to add a **vehicle** to an active ingredient to provide a **final volume** when preparing a solution or suspension. For example, to prepare an oral suspension, the powder is placed in a graduated conical cylinder and distilled water or syrup is stirred into the powder in small amounts until the required volume is reached. Glassware with "to measure" markings are used to accurately measure components of a formulation, such as measuring 1 mL of a flavoring agent that will be added to an oral liquid.

A **beaker** is a straight-sided glass vessel. A beaker may have "to make" or "to measure" markings and range in size from 5 or 10 to 1000 mL or more (Figure 3-5). **Graduated cylinders** are also straight sided, but the markings on a graduate are usually in smaller units of measure, often 1 mL (Figure 3-6). The equal diameters of the graduate from top to bottom, combined with the smaller unit markings provide "to measure" accuracy. **Conical cylinders** are wider at the top than at the bottom (Figure 3-7). Conicals are considered "to measure" glassware. In general, graduates are used to measure ingredients and conicals are used to measure the final volume of the preparation. While a balance is used to measure material by weight, beakers, graduates, and conicals measure volume. Weight is generally a more precise measurement than volume, but often one measurement informs the other. We will clarify this statement as we discuss the different dosage forms in later chapters of this text.

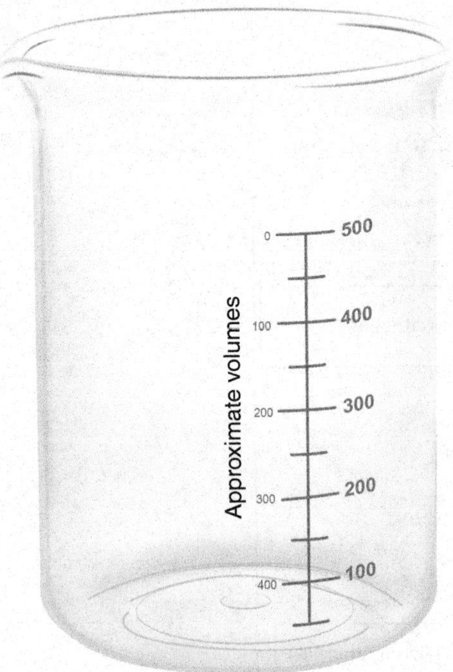

FIGURE 3-5 Beaker.

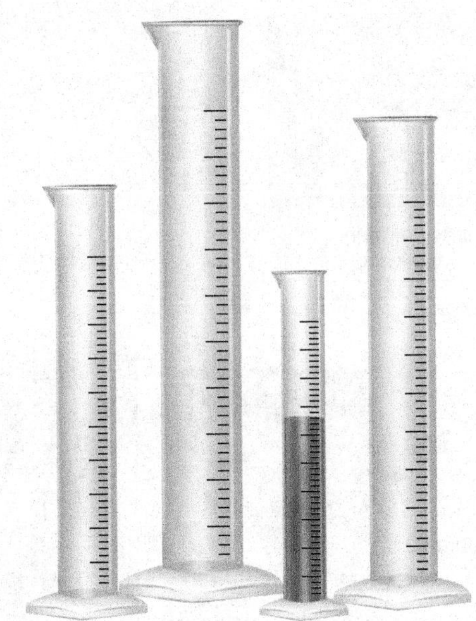

FIGURE 3-6 Graduated cylinders.

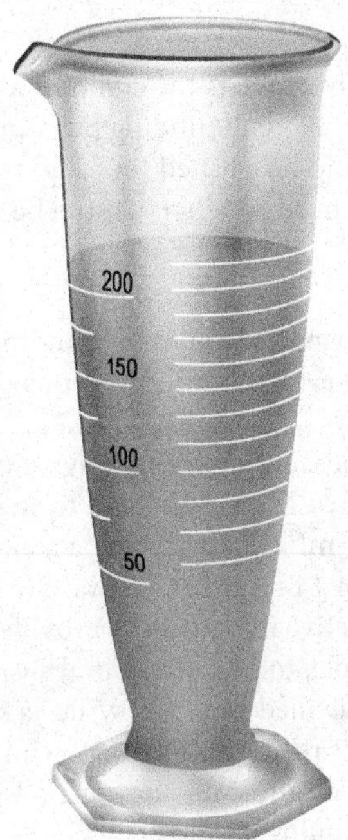

FIGURE 3-7 Conical cylinder.

Mortar and Pestle Sets

It is imperative that the compounding area be equipped with an ancient tool of compounding, the **mortar and pestle (M&P)**. A mortar is a bowl-shaped vessel and a pestle is a shaped rod. The pestle has a handle end and a rounded, stirring end that fits the mortar it matches. Mortar and pestle sets are available in various sizes, as small as 2 oz and as large as 32 oz. Be sure to use a matching set to ensure that the outside curve of the pestle fits perfectly with the inside curve of the mortar. For example, use a 4 oz pestle in a 4 oz mortar.

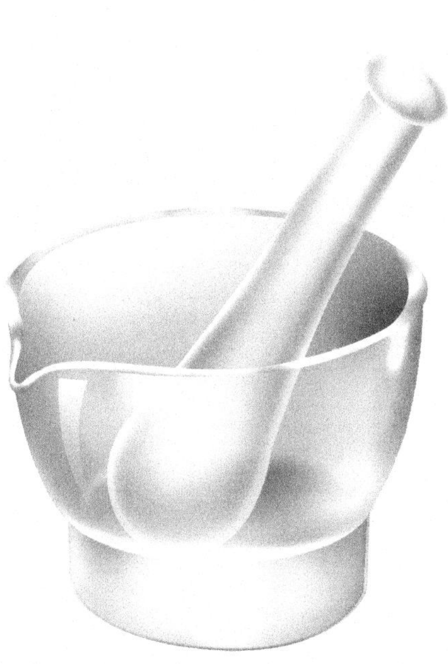
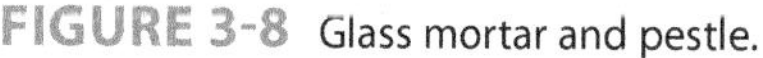

FIGURE 3-8 Glass mortar and pestle.

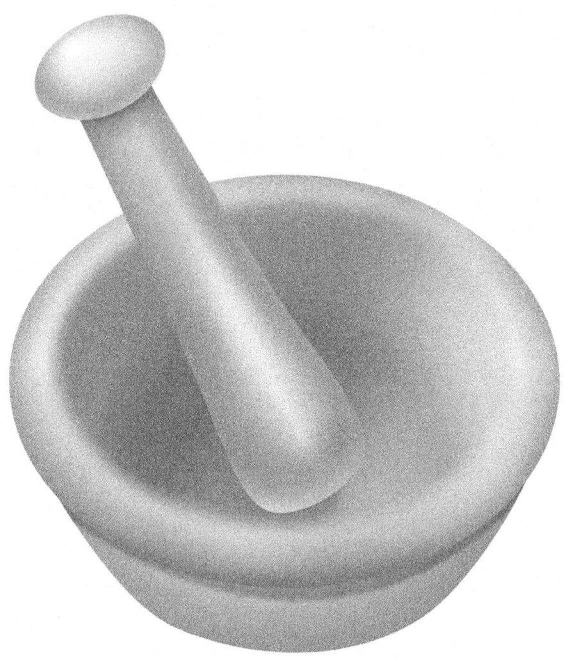

FIGURE 3-9 Porcelain mortar and pestle.

The most common mortar and pestle sets are made from either a porcelain material or of glass (Figure 3-8). The glass is heavy like a beer mug or bar tumbler, and the surface of both the mortar and pestle are smooth. Porcelain mortar and pestle sets are made of porcelain clay and glazed with a white ceramic coating (Figure 3-9). The inside surface of the ceramic mortar is rough as is the mixing end of the pestle.

Glass mortar and pestles should only be used to *combine* ingredients used in non-sterile compounded preparations.

Porcelain mortar and pestles are used to crush tablets and reduce particle size.

Mortar and pestle sets are used to perform two basic functions: **triturate** particle size of powders and create **gross mixtures**. Because of the rough surface on the inside of the mortar and of the shaped end of the pestle, a ceramic mortar and pestle set is the correct tool to reduce the particle size of a single powder or to reduce the particles of more than one powder to equal size. A ceramic mortar and pestle should also be used to crush tablets. Glass does not produce enough friction between the mortar and pestle to properly reduce the size of particles. The glass mortar and pestle should only be used to combine ingredients that have already been prepared and are ready to be added to the compounded medication. It is important for a technician to remember this distinction in order to create the best quality product for the patient.

Spatulas, Ointment Pads, and Slabs

There are a variety of spatulas that may be used to prepare compounded medications. Traditional **spatulas** are made of stainless steel. Stainless steel spatulas usually have wooden handles. They come in a variety of sizes and are most often used to make creams and ointments by hand. This process is called "spatulation" and is discussed in Chapter 7, with detailed discussion on the preparation of creams and ointments. A stainless spatula is also used to "trim" solid dosage forms like troches. This procedure is discussed in Chapter 6. Some chemicals react to stainless steel, and a hard plastic spatula must be used when compounding these reactive materials. Although these types of spatulas are a standard tool of compounding, sometimes the best tool for the job is a good kitchen spatula. A rigid spatula used to prepare a cream is probably not useful for removing every bit of a preparation from the mortar. A more flexible rubber or silicon spatula found at any kitchen supply store may work best for this and other compounding activities (Figure 3-10).

Spatulation to combine the **active pharmaceutical ingredient (API)** and the vehicle can be performed on a clean counter, an ointment slab, or parchment paper. **Ointment slabs** are made of glass and are available in a variety of sizes. The standard ointment slab is 12 inches × 12 inches and ¼ in thick (Figure 3-11). A heavy duty ointment slab will be ¾ of an inch thick. The slab is placed on the counter and can easily be moved to the sink after compounding

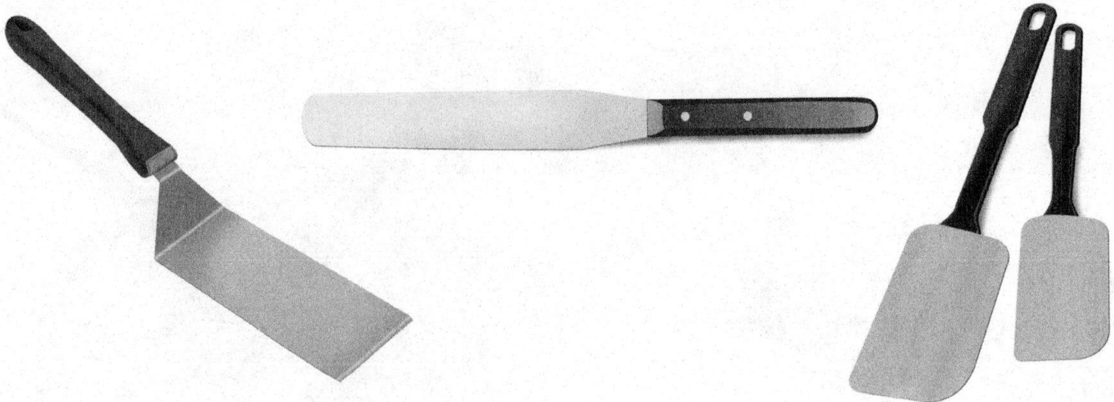

FIGURE 3-10 Examples of spatulas.

FIGURE 3-11 Ointment slab.

for easy clean up. Remember to wash the ointment slab after each compounded product is prepared to prevent cross contamination. Ointment paper, also known as *parchment paper*, can be used in place of an ointment slab. After the cream or ointment is prepared and packaged, the paper is simply discarded. If parchment paper or an ointment slab is not available, ointments and creams can be prepared on a clean counter that is free of blemishes and cracks.

Other common compounding utensils include stirring rods, measuring spoons and cups, sieves, forceps, and more.

Containers and Dispensing Devices

Special bottles and closures also need to be on hand to contain compounded preparations for dispensing. The pharmacy will need to have a variety of containers for different dosage forms. Listed here are some of the dispensing supplies needed:

- Tablet and capsule *vials* with child proof lids
- *Oval bottles* with child-proof lids to dispense liquids
- *Ointment jars* and *tubes* for dispensing creams and emollients
- *Special metered dose containers*
- *Vials* with droppers, brushes, or rods attached to the inside of the caps used to dispense various topical liquids
- *Oral syringes* that are normally used to measure liquids and can also be preloaded with measured doses of creams and gels
- *Applicators* used for insertion of vaginal creams or suppositories
- *Foil papers* used to wrap suppositories and divided boxes to contain them after they are wrapped

Choosing the proper dispensing device is very important to delivering an accurate dose. These devices must have complete and easy-to-follow directions in order to promote patient compliance and ease of use. The proper container is an important part of the preparation and must be on hand in order to complete filling of the prescription (Table 3-3).

TABLE 3-3 Example Containers and Dispensing Supplies

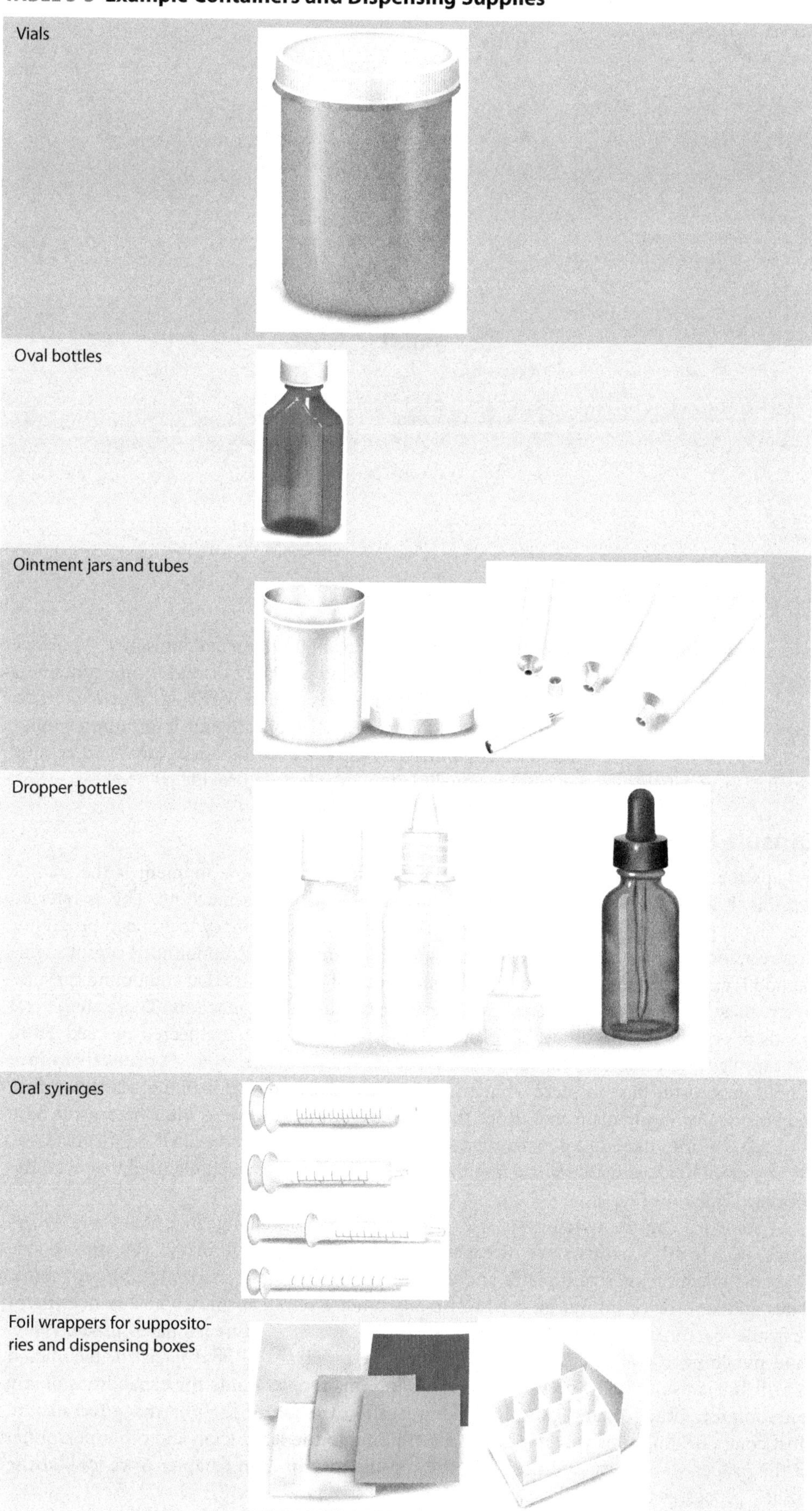

Vials	
Oval bottles	
Ointment jars and tubes	
Dropper bottles	
Oral syringes	
Foil wrappers for suppositories and dispensing boxes	

TABLE 3-3 Example Containers and Dispensing Supplies (*Continued*)

Vaginal and rectal dispenser/ applicators	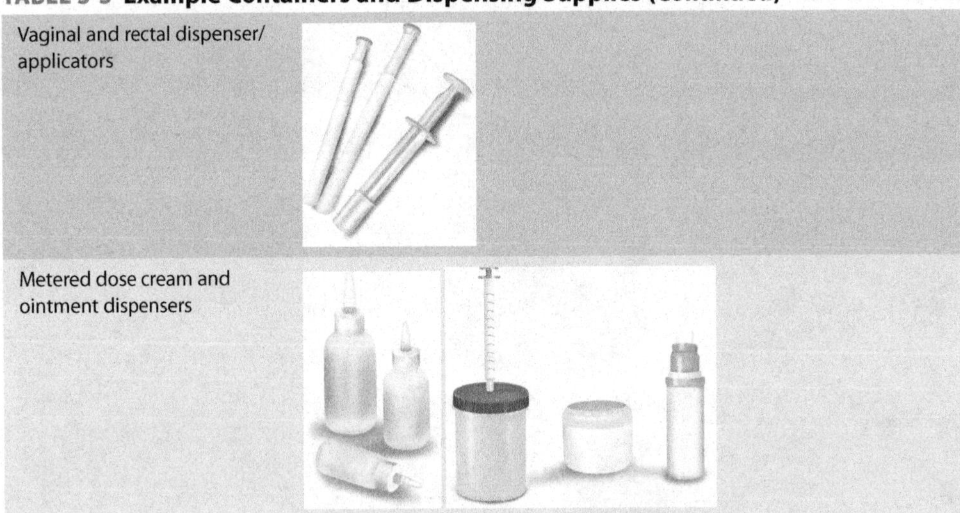
Metered dose cream and ointment dispensers	

SPECIALIZED EQUIPMENT

In its simplest form a compounding area must have certain fundamental tools in it. A balance is required, but a mortar and pestle, a few spatulas, and a supply of dispensing containers may be all that is needed to meet the compounding demand in a particular practice or site. However, many compounding and institutional pharmacies branch out into more complex dosage forms that require specialized equipment. These can benefit patient care by increasing the number of patients serviced and the quality of the medication provided.

Capsule Filling Machines

Perhaps the best example of this need for a specialized piece of equipment is the *capsule machine*. It is possible to fill accurately dosed capsules without a machine. This is referred to as "hand punching" and the technique is taught in many pharmacy technician programs. However, for any pharmacy that requires a substantial amount of compounded capsules, this method is extremely time consuming and inefficient. All pharmacies that compound capsules on a regular basis will usually invest in a precision capsule filling machine. There are several brands of capsule machines available and the most common are engineered to make 50 to 100 capsules at a time. The capsule machine has a stand or base, a set of plates that move to hold the capsule base in place while the capsule cap is removed for filling, and filler plate and an orientor mechanism that drops the capsules into the machine with the capsule base down. Accessories include a powder dam that keeps the powders "corralled" on the machine, a tamper tool to assist with compacting the powders and a special spatula used to spread the powders (Figure 3-12).

A standard capsule machine is size specific or has interchangeable plates and accessories used to fill various sizes of capsules. For example, to fill size 0 capsules, a size 0 capsule machine, or size 0 plates and accessories are required. A size specific machine, plates and accesories cannot be used to fill any other size of capsules. The engineering of a capsule machine is designed to provide ease and accuracy with each batch made. While hand punching 100 capsules could take hours, the experienced pharmacist or technician can fill 100 capsules in 10 or 15 minutes. Having this tool expands the capabilities of any compounding practice, and capsule making is often the job of the pharmacy technician. Most compounding sites will give hands-on training to the technician and other personnel on the proper way to use and maintain the capsule machine. In Chapter 6 we look at the specific processes used to fill capsules.

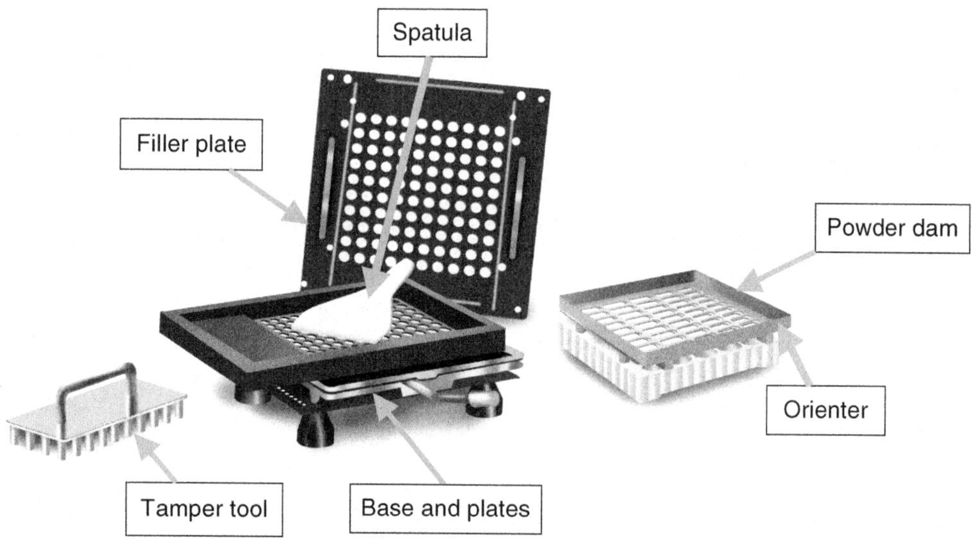

FIGURE 3-12 Capsule filling machine.

Powder Hoods

The powders used in compounding have very fine particle size and many are active, prescription drugs. Each time a container of powder is opened, minute particles of powder escape from the container. Each time a powder is reduced in an M&P, powder is also released into the air. These may be tiny amounts, but over time those powders can be present throughout the pharmacy environment. In addition, these tiny powder particles may fall on the skin or into the eyes, or be inhaled through the mouth or nose of the compounder. Over time, the accumulation of powders could even reach the bloodstream. Many compounding sites invest in a powder hood designed to provide a powder-free environment for their staff and patients (Figure 3-13). The **powder hood** is a counter height box with three closed sides and open front. A fan draws the air inside the hood away from the open front side and into a HEPA filter, or a set of filters. The filtered air is then returned to the room or vented out of the building.

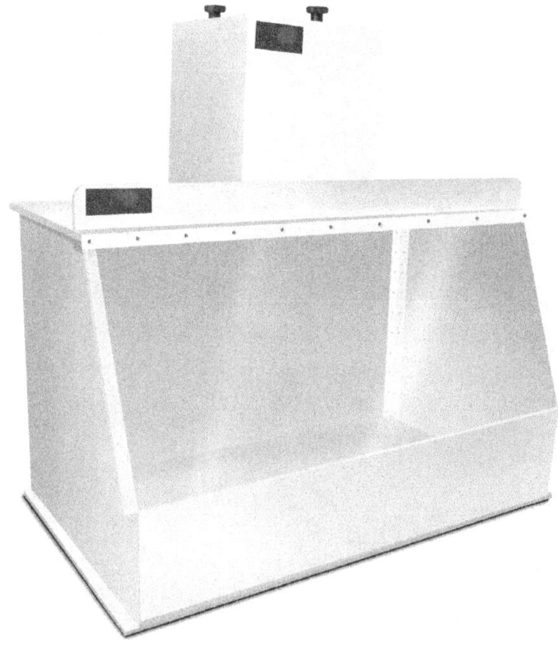

FIGURE 3-13 Powder hood.

MOLDS

Molds are used in the compounding pharmacy to prepare solid dosage forms such as **suppositories**, **troches** (**lozenges**), **lollipops** (lozenges on sticks), gummi chews, and tablets (Table 3-4).

TABLE 3-4 Molds Used in Compounding

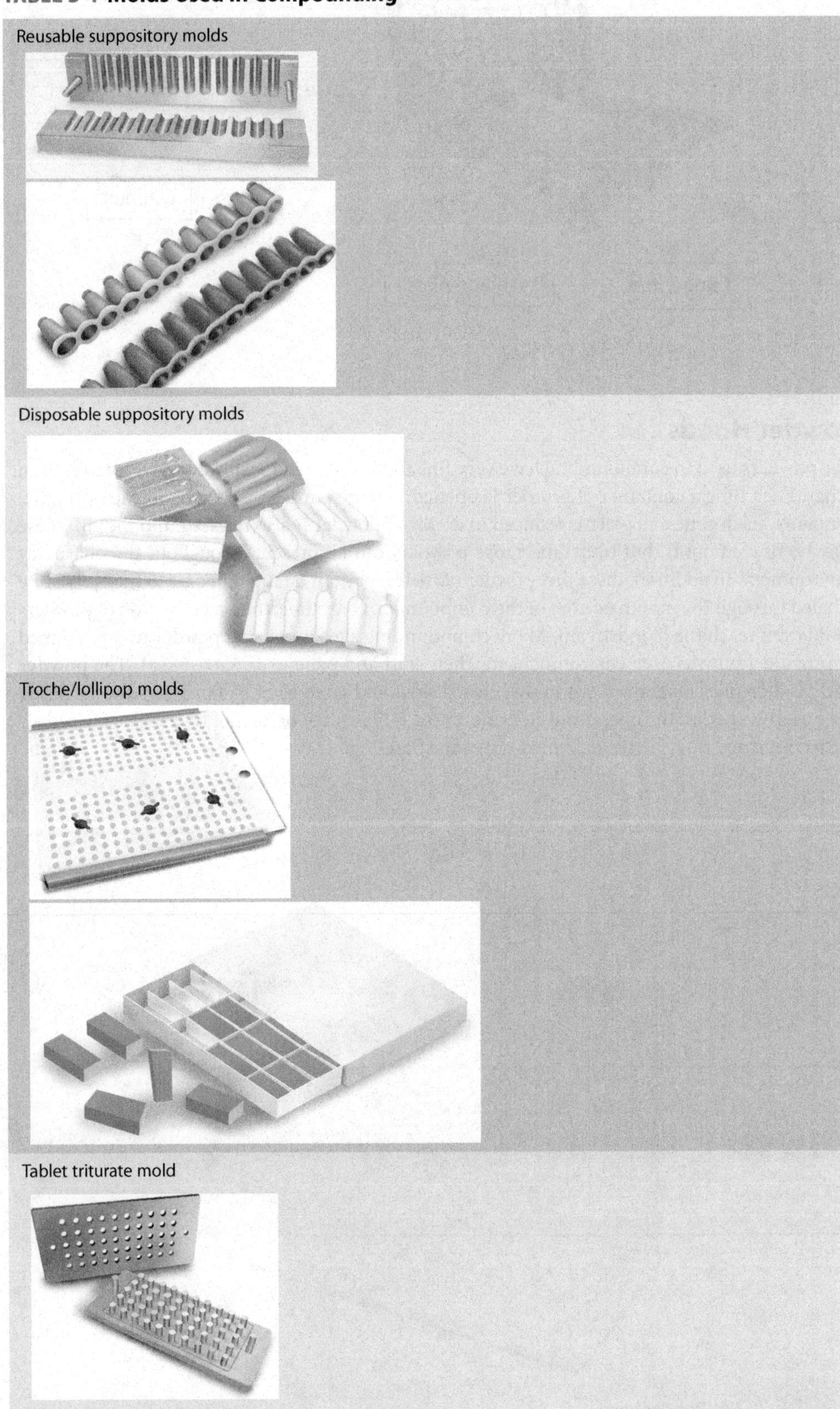

Suppository, Troche, and Lollipop Molds

Molds can be either reusable or disposable. Reusable molds are usually made of aluminum (which are often coated with a nonstick finish) or of a composite plastic material. As with capsule machines, reusable pharmaceutical molds are engineered so that each **cavity** holds a specific volume and can be taken apart for easy cleaning. Formulated material is poured or pressed into the mold, then removed from the mold to be packaged and dispensed. Some molds expand to provide a greater number of cavities, allowing for an increased amount of product to be prepared. Disposable molds are also tooled to provide calibrated cavities; however, the molded dosage forms are dispensed right in the mold and removed by the patient or caregiver when they are administered. There are advantages to both reusable and disposable molds, which include cost, packaging considerations, and patient and care giver convenience (Table 3-4).

Tablet Molds

Tablets are a prime example of the distinction between manufacturing and compounding that was discussed in Chapter 1. Traditional compounding pharmacies that prepare and dispense tablets to an individual patient usually use a mold, while a manufacturing facility would make thousands of tablets using a **tablet press**.

Although they are considered a complex and unique dosage form, two forms of tablets are frequently prepared in compounding pharmacies. **Tablet triturates (TTs)** are tiny **sublingual** dosage forms and **rapid dissolve tablets (RDTs)** are placed on top of the tongue for immediate dissolution. Both of these tablet types are prepared by pressing the tablet material containing the dose of active drug into a calibrated mold (see Table 3-4). Tablets and other solid dosage forms are discussed in Chapter 6.

HEATING AND MIXING DEVICES

A pharmacy that prepares numerous prescriptions every day for liquids, creams, ointments, gels, and lotions often uses specific devices for stirring and mixing compounded products.

Stirrers and Hot Plates

Most products can be stirred manually; however, an electronic magnetic stirring device is less labor intensive, and can save valuable time. A magnetic stirrer has a flat surface that holds a beaker containing a liquid preparation (Figure 3-14). Under the surface there is a rotating magnet powered by an electric motor. A device called a *stir bar*, which is metal rod or crossbar covered in plastic coating, is placed inside the beaker (Figure 3-15). When the motor is turned on, the magnet rotates and spins the bar which stirs the liquid. The speed of the rotation can be decreased or increased from the control knob on the device.

A hot plate is used in a non-sterile setting to melt vehicles for the preparation of solid dosage forms like suppositories and troches. It can also apply the heat necessary to put powders into solution and to melt bases. Hot plates have a single control knob used to regulate the temperature and can be adjusted to provide the high temperatures needed to boil a liquid or the low temperatures used to dissolve chemicals into solution (Figure 3-16).

Some devices combine both of these functions. Stirring hot plates have two control knobs: one to adjust the temperature and the other to adjust the speed of the stirrer (Figure 3-17). The temperature knobs on these devices are often calibrated to indicate the temperature in degrees, and some have digital displays that show the temperature of the heating surface. However, a standard thermometer that will accurately measure the temperature of the material should also be available. A simple glass thermometer inserted into the material in the beaker will verify the temperature reading. There are also electronic thermometers that use a metal probe inserted into the material with a digital temperature display (Figure 3-18). A digital device is often chosen for it durability but either type of thermometer will suffice. *It is important that the thermometer does not touch the sides or the bottom of the beaker as this can cause an inaccurate temperature reading.*

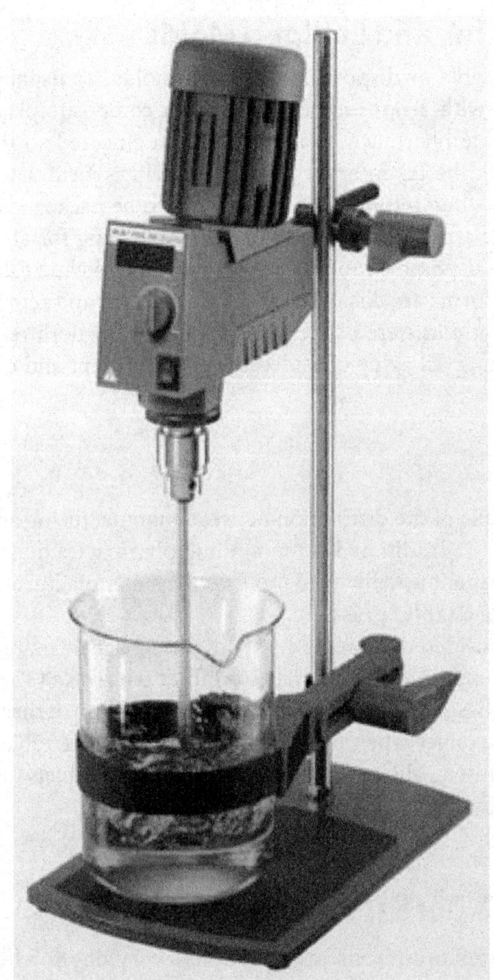

FIGURE 3-14 Electronic stirrer. (*Reproduced with permission from IKA Works, Inc., Wilmington, NC*)

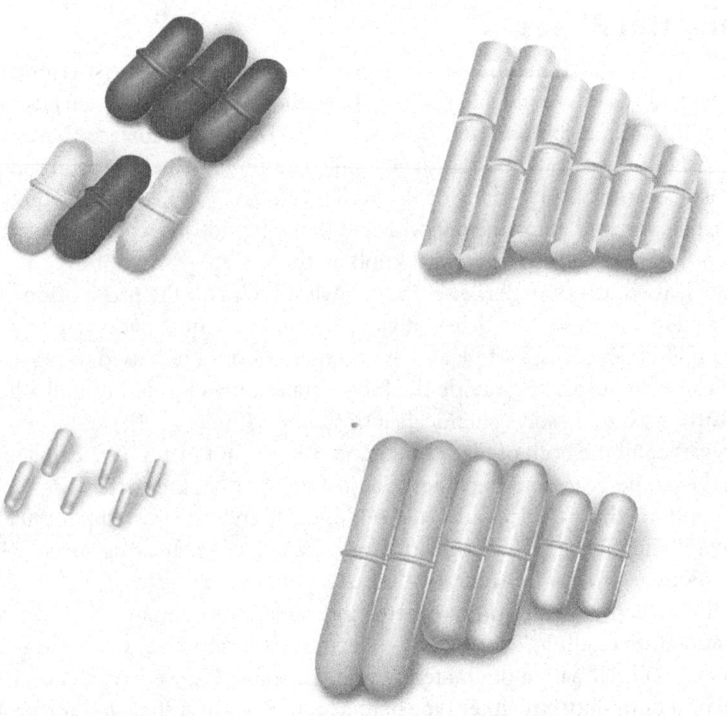

FIGURE 3-15 Magnetic stirring rods.

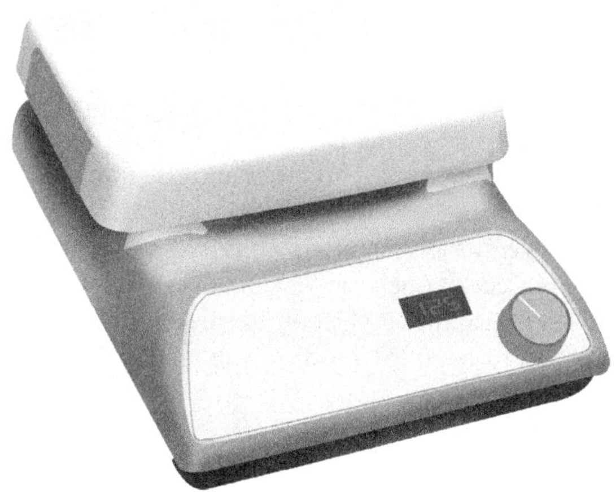

FIGURE 3-16 Hot plate.

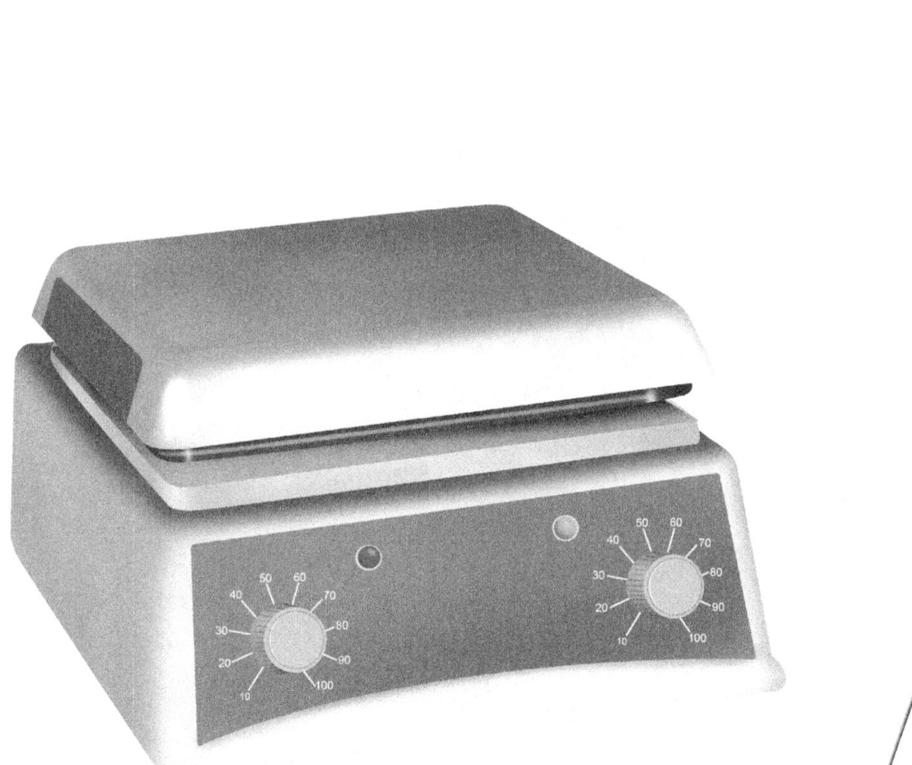

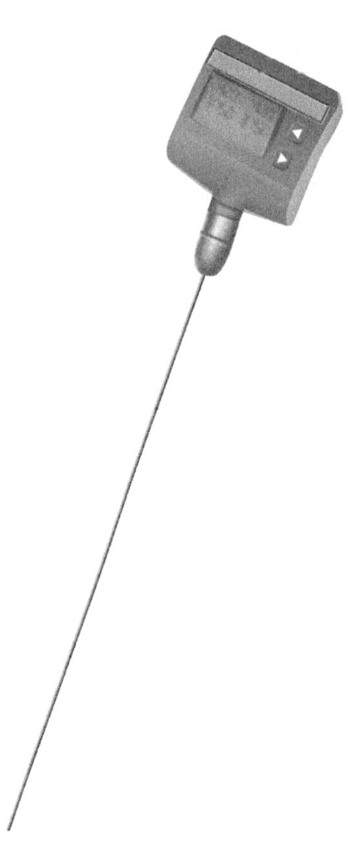

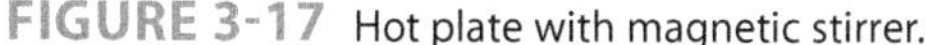

FIGURE 3-17 Hot plate with magnetic stirrer.

FIGURE 3-18 Digital thermometer.

It is tempting to use a microwave oven to melt or heat material being used in a compounded medication, and many pharmacies find them useful. However, every API has a melting point and sometimes that temperature is also the point at which the drug degrades. The actual heat provided by a microwave cannot be measured accurately. In addition, most microwaves provide heat in bursts. While it may be very easy to soften an ointment or a suppository vehicle in the microwave, after the API is added it could be problematic to put the material back in the microwave as there is some risk of heating the API past a safe temperature.

Blenders, Mixers, and Homogenizers

Blenders are frequently found in a compounding practice. A blender has small blades located in the bottom of a container that locks onto a motor base. The blades spin at high speed and draws the material down into them where it is whipped into a **homogeneous** mixture. It has a stainless steel pitcher and is the same type used in a commercial kitchen or restaurant. The stainless material is easy to clean and the motor is more powerful than a regular kitchen blender (Figure 3-19). A homogenizer is a device used to homogenize liquids and creams. It creates emulsions by mixing oils with water at extremely high speeds. Liquids or semisolids are placed in a beaker. The stainless steel wand that is attached to a powerful motor is placed in the mixture to be homogenized. The high-velocity motor turns the inner cylinder of the rod to whip the product into a smooth emulsion (Figure 3-20).

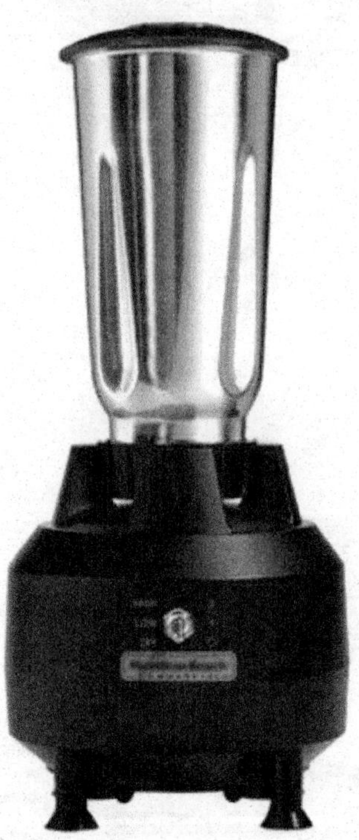

FIGURE 3-19 Blender.

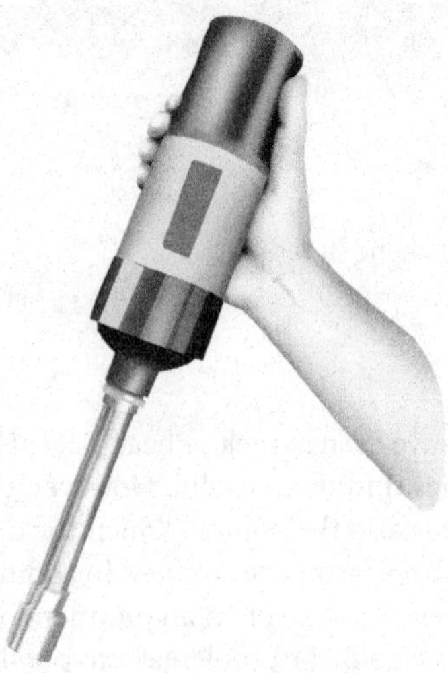

FIGURE 3-20 Homogenizer.

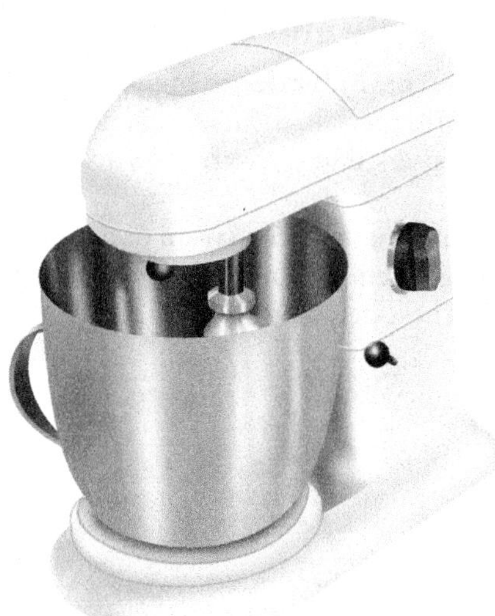

FIGURE 3-21 Tabletop mixer.

Many compounding pharmacies use standard, tabletop mixers to combine ingredients, identical to the one in your kitchen. An industrial-sized floor mixer similar to those used in commercial bakery may be used in a pharmacy that compounds large amounts of a specific product (Figures 3-21 and 3-22).

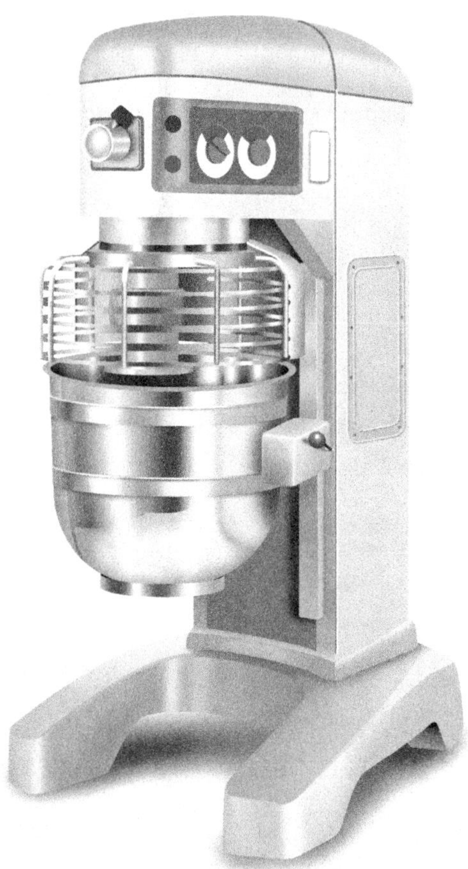

FIGURE 3-22 Floor mixer.

Electronic Mortar and Pestle and Ointment Mills

The **electronic mortar and pestle (EMP)** is a device equipped with a powerful motor, settings for mixing speed and time that uses specialized jars that attach to the machine (Figure 3-23). The jars can also be used as dispensers, and there are a few accessories that allow for even and accurate doses (Figure 3-24).

An **ointment mill** is a machine that moves a cream or ointment through a set of ceramic rollers to thoroughly combine ingredients and reduce particle size, producing a very "finished" looking product (Figure 3-25). These devices are discussed thoroughly in Chapter 7.

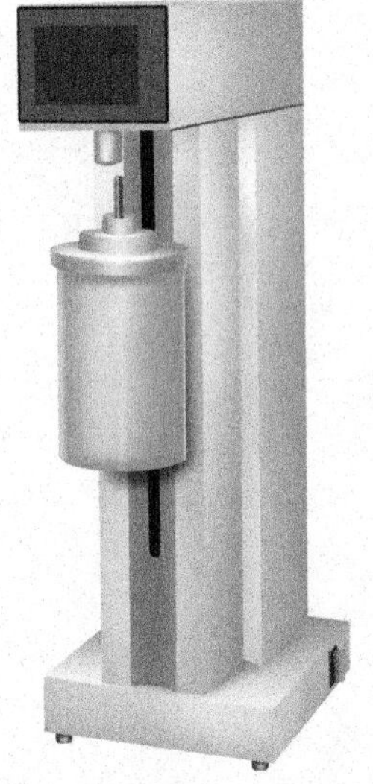

FIGURE 3-23 Electronic mortar and pestle (EMP). (*Reproduced with permission from Unguator Technology.*)

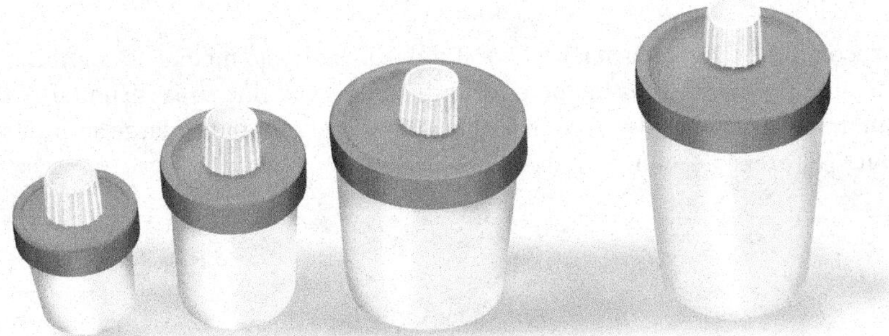

FIGURE 3-24 Dispensing jars used with EMP.

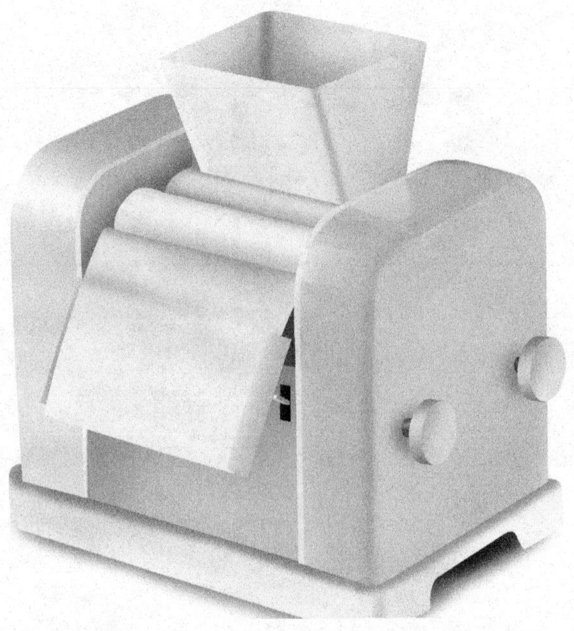

FIGURE 3-25 Ointment mill.

ORDERING AND INVENTORY MANAGEMENT

Based on our discussion in this chapter, there are a various supplies and equipment that are necessary to properly maintain the compounding environment. Pharmacy technicians are often the personnel responsible for making sure devices are kept in working order, and supplies are on hand for use at the non-sterile compounding site. A technician that provides efficient inventory and supply management is a valuable asset to the compounding pharmacy practice.

Supply management may require a daily inventory be taken, or a "want book" that is accessible to staff so they may request items that are running low. Often, **minimum reorder levels (MRLs)** are put in place for disposable supplies. These items are checked regularly to ensure the pharmacy has stock on hand at all times.

Testing of electronic devices to ensure they are working properly must be performed on a regular basis, often at the beginning of each shift and the results must be documented. Inaccurate calibration, faulty equipment, or lack of supplies can cause a delay in a patient receiving necessary medications. Make sure you are familiar with your compounding sites ordering and inventory control practices, and are diligent in requesting needed supplies.

Good inventory and device management increases efficiency and is essential to providing a quality compound in a timely fashion, thus increasing positive patient outcomes and quality of care.

CONCLUSION

The chapters ahead discuss the specific processes involved in preparing each type of non-sterile formulation. A solid understanding of the equipment and tools used to create these medications is an important first step. A pharmacy technician who is proficient in the maintenance and use of compounding equipment and can efficiently manage inventory is a valuable resource to any non-sterile compounding pharmacy environment.

CHAPTER SUMMARY

- All pharmacies must have a working class A balance.
- An electronic balance is the modern standard of practice.
- A scientific balance reads 3 places to the right of the decimal point.
- An analytical balance reads 4 places to the right of the decimal point.
- Both an analytical balance and a scientific balance are accurate to 20% of the amount displayed.
- Electronic balances are extremely sensitive to air movement.
- The balance must be calibrated regularly to ensure that the weight displayed is accurate.
- All compounding equipment must be cleaned after each use to avoid cross contamination.
- "To make" markings on pharmacy glassware are normally in increments of 5 or 10 mL.
- "To measure" markings on pharmacy glassware appear in increments of 1 or 2 mL.
- "To make" markings are used to add vehicle to an active ingredient to provide a final volume.
- A balance is used to measure material by weight.
- Beakers, graduates, and conicals measure volume.
- Glass mortar and pestles should only be used to combine ingredients.
- Ceramic mortar and pestles are used to crush tablets, reduce particle size, and combine ingredients.
- Spatulation is the combining of materials by continuously heaping them together and smoothing them out using a spatula.

- Use of the proper dispensing device is very important to delivering an accurate dose.
- Capsule machines are size specific.
- Various molds are used in pharmacy compounding to prepare solid dosage forms.
- TTs and RDTs are frequently prepared in compounding pharmacies.
- A powder hood removes powder particulate from the pharmacy environment.
- A hot plate is used to apply the heat necessary to put powders into solution and to melt bases.
- Some hot plates are also stirrers.
- A thermometer is necessary to confirm the temperature of the heated materials.
- A homogenizer creates emulsions by mixing at extremely high speeds.
- An EMP can be used to combine ingredients thoroughly.
- An ointment mill moves a cream or ointment through a set of ceramic rollers.
- Inaccurate calibration, faulty equipment, or lack of supplies can cause a delay in a patient receiving necessary medications.
- Good inventory and device management increases efficiency and quality of care.
- A pharmacy technician with an understanding of the processes necessary to maintain equipment and manage supplies is a valuable resource to any pharmacy environment.

PTCB Review Questions

1. Which type of mortar and pestle is used only for combining ingredients?
   A. Glass M&P
   B. Porcelain M&P
   C. Both A and B
   D. Neither should be used
2. What is the most common type of balance found in a pharmacy that compounds regularly?
   A. Scientific balance
   B. Analytical balance
   C. Both A and B
   D. Neither is the most common
3. Which of the following is a *false* statement?
   A. The balance must be calibrated regularly to ensure that the weight displayed is accurate.
   B. Both an analytical balance and a scientific balance are accurate to 20% of amount displayed.
   C. Electronic balances are not sensitive to air movement.
   D. A scientific balance can be used to accurately weigh 20 mg of powder.
4. Which of the following statements are *true*?
   A. Cleaning procedures and schedules are not necessary for specialty equipment used in the compounding pharmacy.
   B. A scientific balance reads 4 places to the right of the decimal point.
   C. Glass mortar and pestles should be used to crush tablets and reduce particle size.
   D. Both an analytical balance and a scientific balance are accurate to 20% of amount displayed.
5. What device is used to melt vehicles for the preparation of solid dosage forms, or apply the heat necessary to put powders into solution.
   A. Homogenizer
   B. Hot plate
   C. Microwave
   D. Ointment mill
6. Which of the following would be a utensil commonly found in a compounding pharmacy.
   A. Stirring rods
   B. Metal spatula
   C. Forceps
   D. All of the above

7. Which of the following statements is *false*?
   A. "To make" markings on pharmacy glassware are normally in increments of 5 or 10 mL.
   B. "To make" markings on pharmacy glassware appear in increments of 1 or 2 mL.
   C. Faulty equipment or lack of supplies can cause a delay in a patient receiving necessary medications.
   D. A graduated cylinder is normally considered to be "to measure" glassware.
8. Which of the following supplies are commonly used in conjunction with an electronic balance?
   A. Weigh boats and Weigh papers
   B. Calibration weights
   C. Weigh canoes
   D. All of the above
9. Which of the following supplies are not used to prepare solid dosage forms in a compounding pharmacy?
   A. Ointment mill
   B. Suppository molds
   C. TT molds
   D. Troche molds
10. Which of the following is a *true* statement?
   A. Pharmacists are the only personnel responsible for making sure that devices are kept in working order in the compounding pharmacy.
   B. All compounding equipment must be cleaned once weekly to prevent cross contamination.
   C. Good inventory and device management increases efficiency and quality of care.
   D. PPE only protects the compounded product from contaminants, not the compounding personnel.

Techs in Practice: Discussion Topics and Questions

SCENARIO 1

Compounding hormonal preparations can be especially challenging in the pharmacy. Men who have compounded estrogen preps on a regular basis have been known to start developing female characteristics, and women compounding testosterone products have shown an increase in facial hair and other male characteristics.

What steps can be taken in the compounding environment to prevent this?

SCENARIO 2

Squaric acid *n*-dibutyl ester (SANDE) is an API often used in preparations to treat warts. SANDE is a thick liquid that evaporates quickly when exposed to air. It is usually included at 1% or less in a preparation.

Considering these properties of SANDE, what is the most accurate way to measure SANDE?

Lab 1

Using the Internet to find a user manual or guide, write a step-by-step procedure for cleaning one of the devices listed below.

- Electronic balance
- Hot plate with a magnetic stirrer
- Powder hood
- Homogenizer
- EMP

Lab 2

Prepare an easy-to-use inventory list for a compounding pharmacy's disposable supplies.

Calculation Review Questions

1. A compounding pharmacy uses an average of 50 weighing boats each day for the first 10 days of the month, and 23 each day for the rest of the month. (Use an average of 30 days in 1 month for this calculation.)
   A. If this trend continued, what is the minimum amount of weighing boats the pharmacy would need to have on hand each month?
   B. What is the total the pharmacy would use in a year?

2. You need to measure the following API powder amounts for a compound:
   API 1: 0.4 g
   API 2: 0.02 g
   API 3: 1.8 g
   A. What would be the total weight of powders used?
   B. What would the total be of each powder if you needed to make 3 times the amount of the original compound?
3. Prepare 350 g of a 2% lidocaine cream using a 1% lidocaine cream and a 5% lidocaine cream.
   A. What is the total amount of the 5% lidocaine cream needed to prepare the final 2% product?
   B. What is the total amount of the 1% lidocaine cream needed to prepare the final 2% product?
   C. Convert the weight of the total amount 2% lidocaine cream prepared from grams to milligrams.
4. How much 3% hydrocortisone cream and water-washable base is needed to prepare 440 g of 1% hydrocortisone cream?
   A. What is the total amount of 3% hydrocortisone cream needed to prepare the final product?
   B. What is the total amount of water-washable base needed to prepare the final product?

This chapter includes the following PTCE Blueprint Knowledge Areas

Section 1.0-1.4 Strengths/dose, dosage forms, physical appearance, routes of administration, and duration of drug therapy.

Section 2.0- 2.6 Record keeping, documentation, and retention (eg, length of time prescriptions are maintained on file).

Section 2.0-2.11 Infection control standards (eg, laminar air flow, clean room, hand washing, cleaning counting trays, countertop, and equipment). (OSHA, USP/NF Chapter <795> and <797>)

Section 2.0-2.13 Professional standards regarding the roles and responsibilities of pharmacist, pharmacy technicians, and other pharmacy employees. (TJC, BOP)

Section 2.0-2.15 Facility, equipment and supply requirements (eg, space requirements, prescription file storage, cleanliness, reference materials. (TJC, USP, BOP)

Section 3.0-3.1 Infection control (eg, hand washing, PPE)

Section 3.0-3.3 Documentation (eg, batch preparation, compounding record)

Section 3.0-3.5 Selection and use of equipment and supplies.

Section 3.0-3.7 Non-sterile compounding processes.

Section 7.0-7.3 Ordering and receiving processes (eg, maintain par levels, rotate stock).

This chapter includes the following Ex-CPT Test Specifications

Section 1 A-4 Comply with rules and regulations when filling prescriptions.

Section 1 A-6 Maintain a clean work environment in the pharmacy and patient care areas.

Section 1 A-9 Assist the pharmacist in managing inventory by placing, receiving, verifying, and stocking orders.

Section 1 A-11 Maintain proper supplies of prescription vials, caps, bottles, and other supplies.

Section 1 C-7 Properly package prescription medication in child-resistant containers or other approved containers as required.

Section 1 C-8 Comply with professional, state, and federal laws and regulations.

Section 2 A-2 Differentiate among various dosage forms (eg, tablets vs capsules, ointment vs creams, controlled release vs immediate release, parenteral vs oral).

Section 3 B-5 Follow proper record keeping procedures pertaining to the pharmacy.

Section 3 B-6 Follow the pharmacy's quality assurance policies and procedures.

Section 3 D-1 Follow proper compounding procedures for non-sterile products.

Section 3 D-3 Repackage and label unit of use products properly.

This chapter includes the following ASHP Model Curriculum for Pharmacy Technician Training Goal Statements, Objectives, and Instructional Objectives

OBJ 3.4 Use knowledge of site's storage system to efficiently secure the prescribed medications or devices from inventory.

OBJ 3.11 Follow safety policies and procedures in the preparation of all medications.

OBJ 3.13 Package the product in the appropriate type and size of container using a manual process or automated system.

OBJ 10.6 Identify pharmaceuticals, durable medical equipment, devices, and supplies to be ordered (eg, "want book").

OBJ 12.3 Maintain a clean and neat work environment.

OBJ 12.5 Follow manufacture's guidelines in troubleshooting, maintaining, and repairing electronic devices used by the pharmacy in the preparation and dispensing of medications.

OBJ 18.2 Maintain personal hygiene.

Answers to PTCB Review Questions

1. **A**
2. **A**
3. **C**
4. **D**
5. **B**
6. **D**
7. **B**
8. **D**
9. **A**
10. **C**

Answers to Calculation Review Questions

1.
   A. 960 a month
   B. 11520 per year
2.
   A. 2.2 g total
   B. 1.2 g
   C. 0.06 g
   D. 5.4 grams
3.
   A. 262.5 g
   B. 87.5 g
   C. 350,000 mg
4.
   A. 146.7 g
   B. 293.3 g

CHAPTER 4

Compounding Documents

INTRODUCTION

Compounding relies on information known about the drugs being used, clinical evidence that indicates appropriateness for the patient's diagnosis, and specific documentation of how the formulation for the compound was chosen. USP/NF Chapter ⟨795⟩ Monograph on Non-sterile Compounding requires that two primary documents be developed for each compound prepared: the **master formulation record (MFR)** and the **master compounding record (MCR)**. The MFR is like a "recipe" and is used to prepare a specific medication whenever a prescription is received for it. The MCR provides specific information about the actual ingredients and methods used to prepare a particular compound. This chapter explains both these documents in detail and discusses other documents that are required in a compounding practice in order for the pharmacy to prepare safe and effective medicinal compounds for their patients.

LEARNING OBJECTIVES

- Describe and explain the contents and purpose of a master formula record (MFR).
- Explain the importance of differentiating between API products with the same name.
- Define and explain the terms "quantity sufficient" (QS) and "quantity sufficient to reach volume" (QS AD).
- Explain the terms commonly seen in compounding instructions.
- Explain the importance of beyond-use dating (BUD).
- Describe the contents and purpose of the master compounding record (MCR).
- Explain the purpose and content of a policy and procedure manual (P&P).
- Explain the purpose and content of a standards of practice (SOP) document.
- Describe a certificate of analysis (C of A).
- Explain the content and purpose of a material safety data sheet (MSDS).
- Explain the content and purpose of pharmacy logs.

KEY TERMS

Aqueous: Containing water

Beyond-use date (BUD): The date on which any remaining amount of a compounded preparation must be discarded

Buffers: Chemicals that are added to a preparation to prevent changes in the pH

Concentration: The amount of a specified substance in a unit amount of another substance

Course of therapy: The duration of time the patient is to take the medication

Dose: The amount of drug taken with each administration

Fillers: Nonactive excipient materials

Geometric dilution: Adding small or equal portions of one substance to another with thorough mixing between each addition until the total quantity is reached

Levigation: To wet powders to a smooth paste

Master compounding record (MCR): A permanent record of the process, materials, and personnel who prepared a medication from an MFR

Master formulation record (MFR): A permanent document that lists each component of the finished preparation; instructions on how to prepare, label, and dispense; and all references used to develop the formulation

OSHA: Occupational Health and Safety Administration—federal agency of the US government that enforces health and safety regulations in the workplace

Particle reduction: Grinding of powder(s) to be used in a preparation so that the size of all the particles is uniform and as small as possible

Policies and procedures (P&P) manual: A document that states the pharmacies' goals, rules, and instructions on how staff members are to perform their work

Quantity sufficient (QS): An amount of an ingredient needed in a preparation that is not measured precisely

Quantity sufficient to reach volume (QS AD): Adding as much as needed of an ingredient to complete the total volume required

Shelf life: New terminology used to express the BUD of compounded medications

Stabilizers: Nonactive excipients used to protect the active drug

Standards of practice (SOP): Specific instructions on how a particular task is to be performed within the pharmacy practice

MASTER FORMULA RECORD

The USP/NF Chapter ⟨795⟩ on non-sterile compounding requires that a *master formulation record* (MFR) must be on file and available to be reviewed by the state board of pharmacy for all compounded medications. The MFR must include the following:

- The name or *title* of the preparation
- A list of every *ingredient* contained in the preparation
- A list of the *equipment and supplies* used to prepare and dispense the medication
- The *procedure and steps* to be followed for preparing the medication
- *Quality parameters* for assessing the preparation before it is dispensed
- *References* for the formulation content
- *Beyond-use date (BUD)* that is assigned to the medication

Title

The name of the preparation must include the name of the active ingredient(s) as well as their **concentration** in the medication. It must also contain the total volume of the preparation and the dosage form used. The name of the formulation is taken from the prescription (Figure 4-1). The name/title of the MFR for this preparation is *metronidazole 250 mg/5 mL oral liquid.*

Metronidazole 250 mg/5 mL oral liquid

To make 120 mL

Sig: Take 1-2 tsp (5-10 mL) orally daily as directed.

No refills

FIGURE 4-1 Example of a prescription for a compounded oral liquid.

Ingredients

The list of ingredients included in the MFR must include all the materials that is used in the preparation. This includes the following (Figure 4-2):

- Active drug (API)
- Excipients or nonactive ingredients included as **fillers** and **vehicles**
- Chemicals that are included as **buffers**, **stabilizers**, etc

Drug name:	Metronidazole	**Dosage Form:**	Suspension
Concentration:	50 mg/mL	**Shelf Life:**	60 days
Route:	Oral	**Storage:**	Refrigerate or Room Temp
Volume:	120 mL	**Auxiliary Labeling:**	Shake Well; Protect From Light

Ingredients	QS	Quantity	Units
Metronidazole Benzoate Powder		6	g
Ora-Blend (or 1:1 Ora-Plus:Ora-Sweet)	X	120	mL

Directions:

1. Weigh powder and place in a mortar.
2. Add 12 mL of the Ora-Blend and mix to a uniform paste.
3. Continue to add Ora-Blend geometrically to almost final volume, mixing thoroughly.
4. Add enough Ora-Blend to bring to final volume (120 mL) and dispense in amber bottle.

Notes:

- May substitute Ora-Blend Sugar Free with same stability. Metronidazole tablets are not used due to palatability. One gram metronidazole benzoate is equivalent to 625 mg metronidazole base (tablets).

References:

- Allen LV, Erickson MA. *Am J Health-Syst Pharm.* 1996;53:2073-2078.

Reviewed: May 2013; JR/SC

The information provided on this site is only to be used for educational and informational purposes only. It may not be relied upon to direct or provide care to a patient, or to prepare treatments for a patient.This material is not intended as a substitute for retaining and consulting appropriate medical and health care professionals, who remain solely responsible to provide and direct patient care. Be aware that the information contained on this site may not be up to date due to more recent medical developments.The preparation, dispensing, and administration of pharmaceuticals is and remains the responsibility of licensed medical professionals or pharmacists, and may require governmental approvals.The owner and provider of this site disclaims and assumes no liability for any injury and/or damage to persons from use of any information contained on this site.

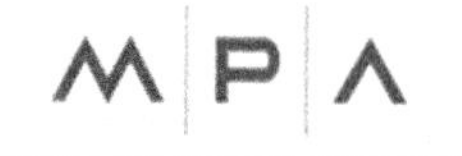

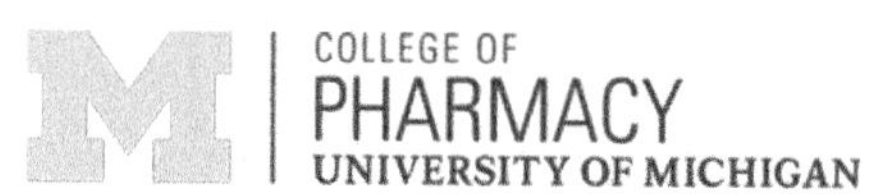

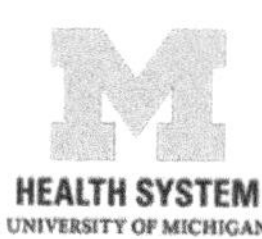

FIGURE 4-2 Example of master formula record (MFR). (*Reproduced, with permission, from the University of Michigan College of Pharmacy. http://mipedscompounds.org. Accessed April 8, 2014.*)

TABLE 4-1 Differences in Lidocaine

Product	Soluble in Water	Soluble in Ethanol	MW
Lidocaine USP	Insoluble	Soluble	234.34
Lidocaine HCl USP	Soluble	Insoluble	270.80

Many active pharmaceutical ingredients have different forms that may start with the same sequence of letters or product name; a good technician knows how important these product differences are in correctly creating the MFR and accurately preparing a compounded prescription medication. Many APIs are available as "base" and "salt" forms. For example, lidocaine has 2 chemical forms that are frequently used in compounding: *lidocaine USP* (often called *lidocaine base*) is the original "compound" of the drug; *lidocaine hydrochloride USP* (*lidocaine HCl*) is the hydrochloride "salt" form of the drug. The primary differences of these 2 active pharmaceutical ingredients are their solubility and molecular weight (MW) (Table 4-1).

Very often, the physician just writes "lidocaine" on the prescription. The pharmacist chooses the drug form to be used in the formulation based on several factors, including solubility; the dosage form to be dispensed; and how the drug is to be absorbed, metabolized, and excreted by the body. The choice between lidocaine USP and lidocaine HCl must also take into account the vehicle to be used. Based on Table 4-1, if the vehicle is water-based, we know that to create a solution, the lidocaine HCl must be used because it is water soluble. For a solution using alcohol as the vehicle, the lidocaine USP base would be used. If the prescription said only "lidocaine," and lidocaine HCl is chosen based on its solubility in water, a conversion must be calculated to provide the proper amount of lidocaine called for in the prescription. Lidocaine HCl has extra molecules in it that are *not* in lidocaine USP, which accounts for the difference in molecular weights. This means that in order to provide 1 g of lidocaine from lidocaine HCl powder, 1.16 g of lidocaine HCl must be measured for each 1 g of lidocaine USP needed in the medication. A good technician recognizes the difference in name in order to calculate the correct amount of API for the formulation.

Many compounding ingredients have similar names; always pay attention and double check that the correct ingredients are used.

Alcohol is another example of a product with many name variations that are used frequently in compounding. For example, *alcohol USP, ethyl 200 proof* is a consumable material, but *alcohol USP, denatured 200 proof* cannot be swallowed without severe harm to the patient. *Consumable alcohol* must be used as a vehicle for oral liquid preparations, but it can also be used to compound creams. *Denatured alcohol* (not consumable) may be used in a cream but *never* in an oral liquid. When reading or creating the MFR, make sure to double-check the formulation for the correct name of the ingredients that are required.

Equipment and Supplies

The MFR should specify which piece of equipment is to be used in the preparation of the medication being dispensed. For example, an ointment mill can not only combine ingredients, it can also reduce the particle size of powders used in a compound. An electronic mortar and pestle (EMP) does not reduce particle size although it is an excellent mixing device. Therefore, while the EMP is an appropriate tool for many things, the mill may be the best choice. Using the same equipment each time a specific compound is made increases the uniformity of the subsequent preparations based on that MFR.

It is important to list each specific piece of equipment in the MFR to assist in troubleshooting if a problem occurs. For example, if the pharmacy has 3 electric balances, they should each have a separate identifying name or number. The MFR for a preparation will list "balance," and when the technician documents the compounding process for a specific preparation on the MCR, they will list the *name or number of the balance used.*

Supplies needed for proper dispensing must also be included on the MFR. Disposable suppository molds are used both to form the suppositories and are also dispensed to the patient as packaging for the medication. Suppository foils are used to wrap the individual suppository when a reusable mold has been used. Listing these supplies in MFR ensures that compounding personnel know exactly which materials will be needed to properly prepare and dispense the patient medication.

Procedures

The procedures listed on the MFR are step-by-step instructions on how the compound should be prepared and the order in which the steps are performed. Some of the fundamental instructions and common compounding terms that a technician must understand and be able to perform properly are listed in this section.

Particle reduction is an instruction that tells the compounding personnel to crush the active medication (tablets or API) into uniform-sized particles.

Geometric dilution is another basic term used to describe a specific technique of mixing active drug into a compounded vehicle. The process begins with the amount of the smallest ingredient, (usually the API), being mixed thoroughly and evenly into the same amount of another ingredient, such as the vehicle. This is done by adding and mixing small amounts of the vehicle into active pharmaceutical ingredient. Then add the same amount of the vehicle as the first mixture and mix again, repeating the steps until the entire required amount of vehicle has been added. Geometric dilution provides even distribution of the API throughout the vehicle.

Levigation is a term used to describe the combining of a powder and a liquid. Often, the MFR instruction states "levigate to a smooth paste." Through the process of levigation, all particles of the powder become completely wet so that when they are incorporated into the vehicle, the powders do not clump together. Unless the powders are evenly distributed throughout the vehicle, 1 **dose** could contain a "clump" of active powder, which would mean the patient received too much drug in 1 dose and not enough in another.

Quantity sufficient (QS) appears as a quantity on the ingredient list of the MFR. This means that the ingredient should be added to the preparation in the required or needed amount, but that the amount might be different depending on circumstances. For example, a flavoring agent is often listed as QS. Maybe 2 different patients are prescribed the same metronidazole 250 mg/mL compounded oral liquid. One patient finds the preparation much more palatable when 2 drops of chocolate concentrate are added. The other patient finds the solution a bit salty, so after checking the MFR, the pharmacist adds a third drop of chocolate concentrate. Because the direction was QS, either amount added is acceptable.

QS AD is an abbreviation for the Latin words meaning **quantity sufficient to reach volume.** QS AD is always the most accurate way to determine the quantity of the vehicle being used. For example, Figure 4-2 lists as ingredients *250 ml of Ora-Blend*, or an *Ora-Plus and Ora-Sweet.* In Step 4 we are instructed to "add enough Ora-Blend to bring to final volume to 120 mL." This instruction could also be written as "QS AD to 120 mL." Both orders instruct the technician making the preparation that the powder (metronidazole benzoate powder) takes up some space in the total volume and that there will be some vehicle remaining when volume is reached. QS AD is used to ensure that the total prescribed volume is not exceeded, so the concentration of the active ingredient is accurate in the final product.

> **QS: "Quantity sufficient."**
> **QS AD: Quantity sufficient to reach volume."**

Figure 4-3 shows an example of how these important terms appear and are used in an MFR.

Packaging and Labels

The packaging used to dispense compounded prescriptions and the labels applied to those packages is essential to the proper use of the medication by the patient. Several factors must be considered to provide the easiest method of administration. These factors may include a patient's age and physical condition, as well as living situation and daily activities. For example, an elderly patient may not have the dexterity needed to open a bottle or measure a liquid dose, or a child might need to be dosed at school by someone other than the primary care giver.

A label must contain the name of the medication, and the name must match the MFR name. It must contain the dosage amount and frequency, and the BUD. It must clearly state storage conditions, and special directions such as "shake well," or "take with food." Any compounded prescriptions dispensed to a patient in a retail pharmacy must have a standard pharmacy label with a prescription number. An institutional pharmacy may prepare a larger amount of various compounded formulations to be kept in the pharmacy for dispensing to individual patients. Both the bulk product and the individual patient dose must be labeled properly to ensure everyone is aware of the contents of the compound.

AMLODIPINE SUSPENSION 1 mg/mL ***Available* commercial *product*: *Amlodipine* 5 mg *tablets*** **Total Prepared Volume = 250 mL suspension**	
Ingredients: Fifty amlodipine Tablets (5 mg/Tab) 250 mL **Ora**-Blend	
Equipment and Supplies Mortar and pestle Graduate	
Compounding Process	
Step 1	In an appropriate mortar and pestle, crush tablets triturate to a fine powder.
Step 2	Add a minimal amount of vehicle and mix well to form a viscous, but smooth and uniform paste.
Step 3	Continue adding vehicle in geometric portions, mixing well.
Step 4	Transfer to graduate.
Step 5	Rinse mortar with vehicle, adding rinse to graduate.
Step 6	**QS AD** to final volume with vehicle. Stir well.
BUD	56 days at room temperature.
References	Nahta MC, Morosco RS, Hepple TF. *J Am Pharm Assoc.* 1999;(39):375-377.
Labeling	Amlodipine 1 mg/1 mL Total Volume- 250 mL
Auxiliary Labels required	Shake well
Quality Check	Final product is a thick, white suspension.
Notes	Substitute vehicle - Ora-Plus/Ora-Sweet (1:1)

FIGURE 4-3 Example of master formula record (MFR) with "QS AD."

Auxiliary Labels

Many pharmacies use auxiliary labels that are preprinted in bright colors with pictures. These labels can save space on the pharmacy dispensing label and are a good way to reinforce important information that the patient and caregivers need to be aware of. The auxiliary labels must never cover the information on the primary label. Affixing these labels is a matter of preference, so it is important to be familiar with the rules established in your practice site (Figure 4-4).

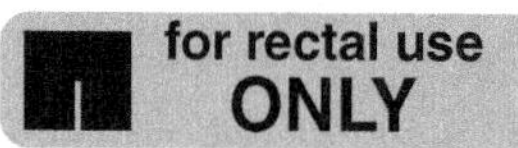

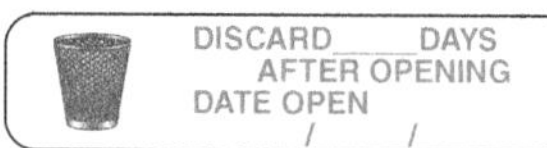

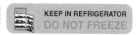

FIGURE 4-4 Auxiliary labels. (*Reproduced with permission from Total Pharmacy Supply, Arlington, TX.*)

Beyond-Use Dates

A beyond-use date (BUD) (also may be expressed as **shelf life**) must be listed in the MFR and applied to each dispensing label. The BUD is the date on which the medication *must be discarded*. The medication is not considered to be safe or effective after that date. The BUD takes into account:

- Degradation of the drug
- The ability of the vehicle to prevent microbial growth

USP/NF Chapter ⟨795⟩ contains a section on how to establish BUD for compounded medications. For example, when two or more manufactured medications are combined, the BUD attached should be the **course of therapy**, or the shortest of the manufacturer's expiration dates found on any API in the formulation. Pharmacists often use a combination of proven BUD from published formulations, manufacturer's product information, and professional judgment to establish BUD for compounded products.

Each compounded medication must be assigned a BUD, and the pharmacist must be able to document a reference for the compounded drug's BUD.

USP/NF Chapter ⟨795⟩ also lists standard BUD for specific dosage forms when *no stability data is available* (Table 4-2).

TABLE 4-2 USP/NF Chapter ⟨795⟩ Beyond-Use Dates for Non-sterile Compounded Formulations Without Stability Data

Formulation	Beyond-Use Dates
Oral formulations prepared in **aqueous** vehicles	14 days, under refrigeration or the earliest expiration date of any component in the formulation, whichever comes first.
Nonaqueous formulations	Maximum of 6 months or the earliest expiration date of any component in the formulation, whichever comes first.
Aqueous topical and *semisolid* formulations	Maximum of 30 days or the earliest expiration date of any component in the formulation, whichever comes first.
Solid dosage forms	The earliest expiration date of any component in the formulation, or a maximum of 6 months, whichever comes first.

A BUD is *not* the same as an expiration date. The active pharmaceutical ingredients and vehicles used in compounding have an expiration date assigned by the manufacturer. A BUD is assigned to a compounded preparation. Both expiration dates and BUD indicate the day on which the material must be discarded. Both are based on stability (the lack of degradation of the material) and storage conditions.

Quality Parameters

Each MFR should also include parameters for how to evaluate the quality of the preparation before it is approved to be dispensed. These can be objective, such as checking the pH level, or subjective, such as recording simple visual observations such as whether the color and texture of the preparation appear uniform throughout the preparation. Suggested quality parameters are often listed in the published formulation that was used as the template for the MFR. Quality parameters serve as a reminder that a close visual examination is the final step in compounding a medication for a patient to ensure that there are no obvious defects.

Notes

The notes section of the MFR should include useful information and/or details about the materials to be used that can benefit any individual preparing the medication, for example the solubility of the active powders, or whether or not another vehicle is acceptable in place of the one listed in the ingredients section (see Figure 4-3). A simple tip in the notes section can save time and prevent errors.

Although the pharmacist is responsible for the calculations and instructions contained in an MFR, a technician often provides "second eyes" that ensure that the information is correct and easy to follow. Experienced technicians can often assist the pharmacist by preparing a "first draft" of an MFR for the pharmacist's approval.

MASTER COMPOUNDING RECORD

The master compounding record (MCR) is a record of the preparation of a specific medication that has been compounded to fill one or more individual prescriptions. This document contains the particular details of each line of the MFR. For each ingredient the actual amount weighed is recorded in the MCR, as is the manufacturer who provided that ingredient to the pharmacy and the lot number of that material. The MCR is where the technician documents which balance was used to measure the ingredients. The MCR should also provide the name of the person who prepared the medication, who performed the QA/QC checks, and who released the preparation to be dispensed.

In addition, the references used to write the MFR and to document the BUD must appear on the MCR. For example, "A BUD of 14-days, refrigerated, may be applied to this preparation" should appear in both the MFR and the MCR for the preparation. The actual *date* (the day, month, and year on which the medication must be discarded, ie, *5/7/14*) must appear on the *dispensing label* and on the completed MCR.

In some pharmacies, a simple photocopy of the MFR is made, and the pharmacist or technician who prepares the medication writes the required information directly on the copy. The copy is now an acceptable MCR. Many compounding practices use software programs that store the MFR electronically and also provide the MCR as an electronic document that can be completed from the keyboard. Regardless of the sophistication of record keeping, both the MFR and the MCR for individual products must be kept and made available for review by the state board of pharmacy. The information in both documents must match. Accurate MCR documents are required to provide easy access to pertinent information that may be needed to identify errors or problems that may have occurred during the compounding process (Figure 4-5).

POLICIES AND PROCEDURES AND STANDARDS OF PRACTICE

Policies and procedures (P&Ps) and **standards of practice (SOPs)** are documents that instruct the manner in which activities in the pharmacy practice are to be performed. These are common in institutional pharmacies such as hospitals and health care centers. Retail pharmacies have recently adopted these types of documents based on new legislative rules by the state board of pharmacy.

Policies and Procedures

Policies and procedures (P&Ps) are global instructions. They include mission statements, organizational charts, employee evaluation and performance standards, benefits and vacation policies, etc.

MASTER Compounding Record

Product Name_______________________________ **(Batch#)**________________

Date prepared :________________ **EXP:**____________________

	Ingredient	Manufacturer	Lot # *	Expiration	Amount	Tech/Rph
1						
2						
3						
4						
5						

	Equipment used	Device#/ Lot #	Manufacturer	Tech/Rph
1				
2				
3				

Compounding instructions:

____

____

____

____

____

____

Labeling:
Drug Name Strength:
Filler:
Amount prepared ____
Date of Prep:____________________
Internal lot
#____________________________
Expiration of Prep'd drug:____________

Reference for formulation:

____

Reference for BUD

____

Theoretical Yield________Actual Yield:________Reason for Discrepancy__________________

Manufactured By:____________Checked by:______________Date:______________

FIGURE 4-5 Sample blank master compounding record (MCR).

P&P manuals in the retail setting guide the behavior of a relatively small staff of workers and are likely to be fairly general. This document may include instructions on how to handle circumstances that might arise, such as billing and payment procedures, or customer relations as well as work schedules and employee evaluation parameters.

In pharmacies located in institutional facilities, the pharmacy will likely follow the P&P manual adopted by the institution. General P&Ps are followed by all employees of the institution, from the laundry to the ICU. The pharmacy has its own policies and procedures in addition to those of the institution. In order to keep institutional certification and licensing, the institutional pharmacy may require more stringent training and recertification of the individuals it employs than are required in a retail pharmacy. Regardless of how brief or involved, every pharmacy practice is required to have a P&P manual that is written in clear, precise language and is accessible to all employees.

Standards of Practice

Standards of practice (SOPs) inform the employees and others how specific tasks are performed in the pharmacy. SOPs should be written for every routine task performed in the compounding area. For example, there should be SOPs for cleaning glassware, calibration of the balance, disposal of materials, and many more. Regardless of how mundane the process might seem, the SOPs should provide step-by-step instructions that can be easily located and understood. Because many of these activities are the same regardless of the type of practice, SOPs may look similar in various settings. Technicians are often tasked with preparing and keeping these documents up to date.

SOPs in the institutional pharmacy may also be written to include staff beyond the pharmacy. For example, the compounding performed by an inpatient pharmacy will probably include interactions between the pharmacy and the nursing staff. Therefore, the SOP would detail how the medication is transferred from the pharmacy to the nursing unit for patient administration. Vendors and suppliers may ask for SOPs regarding drug destruction or purchasing policies. Following these standards will assist the institution in providing quality care for their patients and a pleasant work environment for employees (Figure 4-6).

CERTIFICATE OF ANALYSIS

Each product repackaged by a distributor of materials used to prepare a compounded medication must have a certificate of analysis (C of A). This certificate is a document that lists the USP/NF or other compendia parameters for that material. The C of A is the document that provides the expiration date of the materials in the original container. This document must be examined for accuracy when the product is received, and filed in case of an inquiry from the board of pharmacy or other regulatory bodies (Figure 4-7).

MATERIAL SAFETY DATA SHEETS

A material safety data sheet (MSDS) is not specific to a particular distributor like the C of A, but instead lists information about the material itself, regardless of where it was manufactured. MSDS may be found online at a number of websites, and manufactures or distributors include copies of these documents, or links to online versions, when materials are delivered to the pharmacy. The MSDS informs the individual handling the material of its chemical makeup and details like its molecular weight and solubility. The MSDS also lists proper storage conditions, hazardous material rating, what to do if the material comes into contact with skin, eyes or respiratory system, or if it is ingested accidentally. MSDSs are part of the universal information system and contain international standard labeling requirements. An MSDS for every material used must be on file in the pharmacy. There are MSDSs available at various sites on the Internet.

LOG BOOKS

Log books are used to document recurring activities in the compounding area. For example, log books are kept at each balance, and the daily recording of the calibration of the device is probably one of the duties of the technician working in the compounding area. Cleaning logs are also common for glassware and molds. Log books provide simple accurate documentation that equipment is working properly and that procedures established for quality compounding are being followed by all the staff (Figure 4-8).

Standard of Practice for Intra-institutional Drug Transport from Pharmacy Locations
Intention or Purpose To describe drug storage and transport from central and satellite pharmacy to nursing units.
Definitions Central Pharmacy: Primary location for drug distribution and services pharmacy administration. Satellite Pharmacy: A separate and distinct medication dispensing area within the pharmacy department that is staffed by a licensed pharmacist. Nursing Unit: A separate and distinct patient care location staffed by nursing and other medical professionals, which includes designated, secured areas for patient specific medication storage.
Procedures 1. The central or satellite pharmacy will process individual medication doses and deliver via a pharmacy technician or other pharmacy staff member to the designated, secured area on the nursing unit. Delivery location decisions will be based on patient safety considerations, drug storage requirements, drug preparation and dispensing requirements, anticipated time of day/day of week for dosing, etc. Drug dispensing must be in accordance with institutional policy and procedure, state and federal laws, and TJC standards. 2. Drug deliveries will be performed by a pharmacist or certified pharmacy technician acting under the supervision of a pharmacist. 3. Based on time-motion studies, maximum time for unimpeded movement of personnel between various pharmacy locations is 10 minutes. Allowing for time-of-day and other variables, it is estimated that transport time between satellite locations will not exceed 20 minutes. 4. All pharmacy locations will deliver medications to nursing units hourly from 0800-2300. 5. All pharmacy locations will deliver medications to nursing units at 0300 and 0600. 6. "STAT" and other emergent medications will be delivered directly to nursing staff within 30 minutes from the time pharmacy receives and approves the medication order. 7. The pharmacist will determine the optimal method for transport of medication in order to ensure compliance with all current pharmacy policies.

FIGURE 4-6 Example of pharmacy standard of practice document (SOP).

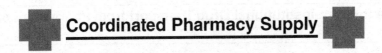

Certificate of Analysis for Empty Gelatin Capsules

Date: OCT 2012 Expiration: DEC 31, 2015

Lot # C432199032 Size: 00 Color: RED 14-091

Physical Characteristics	Unit of Measure	Method	Limits	Real Value
Moisture	%	DCC- MA-P027	13,00-16,00	15,1
Weight	mg	DCC- MI –P003	116,00-130,00	127, 6
Cap length	mm	DCC- MI P006	11,45-12,15	11,62-11,98
Body length	mm	DCC- MI-P006	19,75-20,45	19,96-20,21
Microbiological Limits				
Total viable aerobic count: Bacteria (in cfu/g)	DCC-MA P031	Less than 1000	40	
Escherichia Coli	DCC-MA P036	Negative	Negative	
Salmonella	DCC-MA P039	Negative	Negative	
Staphylococcus A	DCC-MA-P037	Negative	Negative	
Pseudomona A	DCC-MA-P033	Negative	Negative	

Color and Flavor Formulation (% ingredients to 100% gelatin)		
Color -RED	#14-091	This is to certify that all empty capsules manufactured by Coordinated pharmacy supply are made from type B pharmaceutical grade gelatin and meets specifications as described in USP. All ingredients are approved for human use by the US FDA.
Flavoring	Not applicable	
Quality Assurance Rep signature		

FIGURE 4-7 Certificate of analysis (C of A).

Balance Calibration Log

Every week on Thursday use the appropriate weights to determine whether the scale is accurate. For example, place a 0.5 g weight on the scale and if the scale reads 0.5 g then it is calibrated correctly. Write the appropriate weight, date, and initials in the correct box. **Attach balance printout to this sheet. This record should be kept in the front of the Quality Assessment notebook.**

Date	**0.5 g**	**2.0 g**	**10.0 g**	**25.0 g**	**Initials**

FIGURE 4-8 Balance calibration log.

CONCLUSION

Requirements for proper documentation are well defined and must be fulfilled by every compounding practice to ensure patient safety. Each compounded medication must be prepared by following an MFR. The MCR must include the specific lot number of all the materials used in the compound and the name of the vendor or manufacturer for each component must be identified. For each compounding ingredient, a C of A and an MSDS must be on file in the pharmacy and available for review by employees and the state board of pharmacy. In addition, a P&P manual that explains performance expectations must be available to staff. Standard operating procedures must be written and made available to staff so that all compounding activities are performed exactly the same way by all personnel.

CHAPTER SUMMARY

- An MFR must be on file and available to be reviewed by the state board of pharmacy.
- An MFR must include the following:
  - Name or title of the preparation
  - List of all ingredients
  - List of the equipment and supplies used for preparation and dispensing
  - The procedures for preparation
  - Quality parameters
  - References for the formulation content
  - BUD
- The MFR must include all the products that will be used in the compound.
- Many compounding ingredients have similar names but have different properties.
- "QS" and "QS AD" are common terms to describe adding a sufficient amount to accurately complete a compounded product.
- The MFR should specify the equipment and supplies used for a specific preparation.
- The MFR provides step-by-step instructions on how the compounded medication should be prepared.
- A BUD must be applied to each compounded preparation and to the dispensing label.
- The medication is not considered to be safe or effective after the BUD.
- Each MFR should also include parameters for evaluating the quality of the preparation before dispensing.
- Auxiliary labels must never cover the information on the primary label.
- The MCR is a record of the preparation of a particular medication.
- MCR for individual preparations must be kept on file and made available for review by the state board of pharmacy.
- Accurate MCR documents can provide access to information that may be needed to identify errors or problems that may have occurred during the compounding process.
- P&Ps are global instructions.
- SOPs inform employees how specific tasks are to be performed.
- Each product that was repackaged by a distributor and used to prepare a compounded medication must have a C of A.
- An MSDS must be on file in the pharmacy for every material used in compounded preparations.
- Log books provide simple accurate documentation that equipment is working properly and that procedures established for quality compounding are being followed by all the staff.

PTCB Review Questions

1. Which of the following statements are *true*?
   A. An MSDS must be on file and available for review for all products used in the pharmacy.
   B. Auxiliary labels must never cover any information on the primary label.
   C. Both A and B are true.
   D. None of the statements are true.
2. Which document will include chemical makeup and hazardous handling information for a product used in the pharmacy?
   A. MCR
   B. Log book
   C. SOP
   D. MSDS

3. Which of the following must be included in an MCR?
   A. Lot numbers of ingredients used to prepare the formulation
   B. Prescription number
   C. Chemical make up of product
   D. Physician's signature
4. What is *not* included in an MFR?
   A. SOP
   B. Calibration log
   C. Both A and B
   D. BUD
5. What is the pharmacy definition of the term "QS"?
   A. Quality sufficient
   B. Quantity sufficient
   C. Every Sunday
   D. Crush to reduce particle size
6. Which of the following statements are *false*?
   A. The MCR must include the name of the person who prepared the medication.
   B. An MSDS for every material used must be on file in the pharmacy.
   C. C of A is only necessary when products are recalled.
   D. SOPs inform the employees and others how specific tasks are performed.
7. A P&P manual will often include the following:
   A. Organizational charts
   B. Employee evaluation requirements
   C. Employee benefits information
   D. All of the Above
8. Which document will include details on how to perform specific tasks within the pharmacy?
   A. SOP
   B. C of A
   C. MFR
   D. MCR
9. Which document must include the date a particular formulation is prepared?
   A. MFR
   B. MSDS
   C. MCR
   D. SOP
10. Which of the following statements are *false?*
   A. Pharmacists often use published formulation data to determine BUD.
   B. A product is acceptable for use after the BUD.
   C. A BUD must be included on each MFR, MCR, and the dispensing label.
   D. A BUD takes into account the facts regarding degradation of the drug and ability of the vehicle to prevent microbial growth.

Techs in Practice: Discussion Topics and Questions

SCENARIO 1

A cream is put through an ointment mill, and the volume of the preparation increases because the action of the rollers adds air to the cream.What should be added to the notes section of the MFR to alert staff members of this fact?

SCENARIO 2

In small groups or as a class, write an SOP for 2 daily classroom activities. Use the template in Figure 4-5.

Why are SOPs important in the pharmacy?

Can you think of SOPs that you may use every day without thinking about it? In or outside the work environment?

Lab 1

Create an MFR for the oral formulation using the following information and template:

> Spironolactone 5 mg/mL suspension for oral use
>
> Triturate into a fine powder, 40 manufactured Aldactone (spironolactone) 25 mg tablets, then levigate with a little bit of Ora-Plus (or Ora-Sweet) to create a smooth paste. Add the remaining Ora-Plus (total of 100 mL) by geometric dilution until mixed thoroughly. Transfer to an amber bottle and QS with strawberry syrup to 200 mL total. Shake well; suspension is good for 60 days at room temperature.

Formulation Name:

Ingredients:
Vehicle:

Equipment and Supplies

Compounding Instructions

Step 1

Step 2

Step 3

Step 4

Step 5

BUD

References used

Labeling

Auxiliary labels required

Is the MFR for spironolactone missing any information? If so, what information is missing?

Lab 2

Find an MSDS for the following:
70% isopropyl alcohol
Chlorhexidine

- What precautions (if any) are necessary when using these products?
- What steps need to be taken if either of these products is ingested?
- What steps need to be taken if either of these products gets in the eyes?
- Is either of these items flammable?

Calculation Review Questions

1. If 100 g of Aquaphor is added to 100 g of 2% lidocaine, what is the concentration of lidocaine in the resulting mixture?
2. An MFR calls for 100 mg of an active drug powder. This drug is not available as an API so you are instructed to use 20 mg tablets to prepare the compound. How many tablets are needed to equal the 100 mg needed?
3. Seven patients are scheduled to pick up refills of lidocaine 5% ointment in the next week. To save time, the pharmacy schedules making a bulk batch of this preparation which will be divided for dispensing to the individual patients. Each prescription is for 60 g. How much will be prepared to fill these 7 prescriptions?

This Chapter includes the following PTCE Blueprint Knowledge Areas

Section 1.0-1.4 Strengths/dose, dosage forms, physical appearance, routes of administration, and duration of drug therapy.

Section 2.0-2.1 Storage, handling, and disposal of hazardous substances and wastes (eg, MSDS).

Section 2.0-2.2 Hazardous substance exposure, prevention, and treatment (eg, eyewash, spill kit, MSDS).

Section 2.0-2.6 Record keeping, documentation, and retention (eg, length of time prescriptions are maintained on file).

Section 2.0-2.11 Infection control standards (eg, laminar air flow, clean room, hand washing, cleaning counting trays, countertop, and equipment). (OSHA, USP/NF Chapter ⟨795⟩ and ⟨797⟩)

Section 2.0-2.13 Professional standards regarding the roles and responsibilities of pharmacist, pharmacy technicians, and other pharmacy employees. (TJC, BOP)

Section 2.0-2.15 Facility, equipment, and supply requirements (eg, space requirements, prescription file storage, cleanliness, reference materials). (TJC, USP, BOP)

Section 3.0-3.3 Documentation (eg, batch preparation, compounding record).

Section 3.0-3.4 Determine product stability (eg, receptacles, waste streams).

Section 3.0-3.5 Selection and use of equipment and supplies.

Section 3.0-3.7 Non-sterile compounding processes.

Section 5.0 Communication channels necessary to ensure appropriate follow-up and problem resolution (eg, product recalls, shortages).

Section 6.0-6.3 Calculate dosing required.

Section 6.0-6.4 Fill process (eg, select appropriate product, apply special handling requirements, measure and prepare product for final check).

Section 6.0-6.5 Labeling requirements (eg, auxiliary and warning labels, expiration date, patient specific information).

Section 6.0-6.6 Packaging requirements (eg, type of bags, syringes, glass, PVC, child resistant, light resistant).

This chapter includes the following Ex-CPT Test Specifications

Section 1 A-4 Comply with rules and regulations when filling prescriptions.

Section 1 C-8 Comply with professional, state, and federal laws and regulations.

Section 1 C-9 Use information found on medication stock bottles, such as drug name and strength, expiration date, and lot number.

Section 2 B-1 Interpret basic medical terminology used in the pharmacy in order to effectively assist the pharmacist.

Section 2 B-6 Recognize physical interactions and incompatibilities in the preparation of compounded and parenteral medications.

Section 3 B-2 Identify drugs that require special handling procedures.

Section 3 B-5 Follow proper record keeping procedures pertaining to the pharmacy.

Section 3 B-6 Follow the pharmacy's quality assurance P&Ps.

Section 3 B-14 Properly and accurately prepare prescription labels.

Section 3 B-18 Use auxiliary labels properly.

Section 3 B-19 Properly label drug products packaged in approved containers or, when appropriate, original packages.

Section 3 C-2 Calculate the quantities of prescription medications to be dispensed.

Section 3 C-4 Properly calculate individual and daily dosages.

Section 3 D-1 Follow proper compounding procedures for non-sterile products.

Section 3 D-3 Properly repackage and label unit of use products.

This chapter includes the following ASHP Model Curriculum for Pharmacy Technician Training Goal Statements, Objectives, and Instructional Objectives

OBJ 2.4 Efficiently secure information to complete a prescription/medication order.

OBJ 3.3 Follow established laws and protocols to select the appropriate product.

OBJ 3.5 Accurately count or measure finished dosage forms as specified by the prescription/medication order.

OBJ 3.6 Collect the correct ingredients for sterile or non-sterile products that require compounding.

OBJ 3.7 Accurately determine the correct amounts of ingredients for a compounded product.

OBJ 3.11 Follow safety P&Ps in the preparation of all medications.

OBJ 3.13 Package the product in the appropriate type and size of container using a manual process or automated system.

OBJ 3.14 Follow an established manual procedure or electronic procedure to generate accurate and complete product labels.

OBJ 3.18 Follow established P&Ps for recording the preparation of bulk, unit dose, and special doses of medications prepared for immediate or in anticipation of future use.

OBJ 3.19 Follow the manufacturer's recommendation and/or the pharmacy's guidelines for storage of all medications prior to distribution.

Answers to PTCB Questions

1. C
2. D
3. A
4. C
5. B
6. C
7. D
8. A
9. C
10. B

Answers to Calculation Questions

1. 1%
2. 5
3. 420 g

CHAPTER 5

Liquid Dosage Forms

INTRODUCTION

Compounded liquid medications are prepared in most pharmacies, including both hospital and retail settings nearly every pharmacy in this country. Liquid dosage forms provide a precise dose of a prescribed medication in stable, pourable vehicles as either solutions or suspensions. *Non-sterile* (NS) liquid dosage forms can be delivered orally, directly into the stomach, to the skin, or into the rectum or vagina. Liquid dosage forms delivered to the eye, nose, bloodstream, or respiratory system must be compounded under sterile conditions.

LEARNING OBJECTIVES

- Describe non-sterile (NS) liquid dose formulations.
- Explain the difference between solutions and suspensions.
- Explain dilution and reconstitution as they relate to NS compounded liquids.
- Describe the common types of vehicles used to prepare compounded liquids.
- Explain the use of flavoring agents in oral liquids.
- Describe the delivery of oral medications through a G-tube (gastronomy tube) or NG-tube (nasogastric tube).
- Describe and explain topical liquids dosage formulations.
- Describe sublingual drops.
- Describe the use of enemas and douches.
- Describe the 2 forms of a drug that may be used as source-of-drug in a compounded liquid.
- Explain parameters for assigning a beyond-use date (BUD) for compounded liquids.
- Describe products that have special compounding considerations.
- Explain the correct labeling of liquid compounds and the use of auxiliary labels.

KEY TERMS

Aliquot: A portion of material that is too small to be weighed accurately by itself

Alkaline: A pH level greater than 7

Bitterness maskers: Products used to disguise bad tasting medications by adding sweetness to the preparation

Caustic: Able to destroy or burn something by chemical action

Dilution: The process of mixing one material with another that decreases the concentration of the first material. Also, the material created by adding a diluent to a known amount of a material

Distilled water: Water that has many of the impurities removed through distillation that involves boiling the water and condensing the steam into a clean container

Elixir: A liquid containing water and ethanol (ETOH) where the ETOH is included to help dissolve drugs that are insoluble in water alone

Fixed oil: Oil from a plant or animal source, which is nonvolatile and does not evaporate

Fungus: Spore producing organisms feeding on organic matter

G-tube (gastronomy tube): A tube inserted through the abdomen that delivers nutrition and medication directly to the stomach

High-performance liquid chromatography (HPLC): A technique in analytic chemistry used to identify and quantify the amount of each component of the mixture

Inert: Without active properties

Magic mouthwash (MMW): The common name for any number of combinations of medications that are used to treat conditions in the mouth

MDF: Manufactured drug formulation

Miscible: Able to be combined

NG-tube (nasogastric tube): A tube inserted through the nose and throat to deliver nutrition and medication directly to the stomach

Purified water: Synonym for distilled water

Propylene glycol: A liquid solvent commonly used in small amounts in compounded preparations

Reconstitution: To return to a liquid state by adding water

Soluble: Able to be dissolved in a liquid

Solution: A mixture of powder and liquid in which the powder is completely dissolved in the liquid

Stability: The amount of time an active drug retains potency when it is placed in a compounded dosage form. Also refers to the time an aqueous liquid can be expected to not contain microbial growth

Starch NF: Pharmaceutical grade excipient powder, usually derived from corn, which is used as a thickening agent in some structured suspending vehicles

Stevia: A herb used to sweeten sugar-free compounded oral liquids

Structured suspending vehicle: An aqueous vehicle that has been formulated to provide adequate suspension of particles in a compounded oral liquid

Suspension: A mixture of powder and liquid in which the powder is surrounded by the liquid

Swish and spit: Topical route of administration of a liquid substance to the oral mucosa

Syrup: Sweetened water

Wart: A topical irritation caused by a virus

SOLUTIONS AND SUSPENSIONS

Understanding what is meant by the terms solution and suspension and recognizing the differences between these two types of liquids is crucial in choosing the correct vehicle for a liquid dosage form. A **solution** is a mixture of liquid and powder in which the powder is completely dissolved in the liquid. A solution does not require shaking because all of the powder has been absorbed and become part of the liquid.

A **suspension** is a mixture of liquid and powder in which the powder is only surrounded by, or "suspended" in the liquid. The powder particles stay separate from the liquid. A suspension *must be shaken* prior to measuring the dose so that the powders that have settled out of the liquid are redistributed into the vehicle. Without proper shaking, the dose will not contain the proper amount of the active drug.

A suspension must be shaken at the time of administration to ensure the patient is receiving a complete dose of medication.

RECONSTITUTION

Reconstitution is the process of adding a liquid, usually water, to a dry powder to create a specific concentration of a medication. The powder to be reconstituted is provided by a manufacturer in a premeasured amount in a dispensing bottle. The manufacturer's label gives instruction for how much water to add to the powder to produce the final medication concentration. For example, azithromycin for oral suspension includes a preweighed amount of powder, and the manufacture label provides instructions as to the correct volume of water to be added to the powder to provide the labeled concentration and volume to be dispensed. When the prescription is received, the azithromycin container is taken from the shelf, the correct amount of water is measured and added to the container, the bottle is vigorously shaken to mix the powder and water, and the proper pharmacy label is affixed to the container for dispensing (Figure 5-1). *Reconstitution is not compounding.* There is no professional judgment or calculation required to provide the prescribed medication. The pharmacist is simply preparing the commercially available medication to

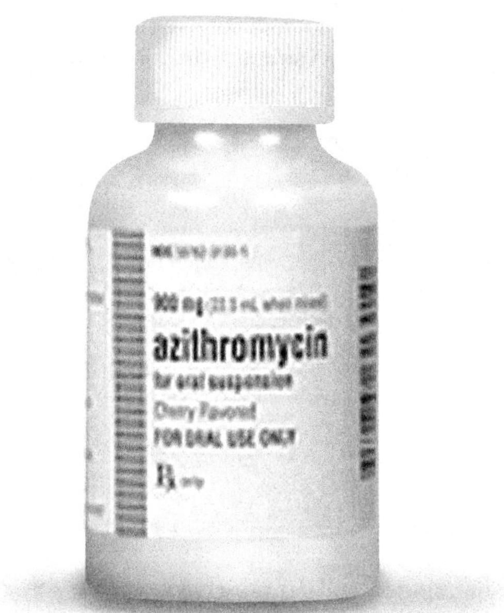

FIGURE 5-1 Azithromycin for oral suspension.

be dispensed. Think of reconstitution as being similar to counting tablets. The pharmacy would not dispense the azithromycin bottle that came from the manufacturer any more than they would dispense the entire bottle of azithromycin tablets that came from the manufacturer. The pharmacy staff must add water in order to dispense the prescribed liquid, just as they must count out the proper number of tablets ordered on the prescription.

DILUTION

If more water is added to a powder for reconstitution than the amount given in the labeled instructions, a **dilution** has been "performed." *Dilution of a manufactured oral liquid is compounding.* For example Tamiflu is provided by the manufacturer at a concentration of 6 mg/mL of oseltamivir. A mother has 3 children that all need to take oseltamivir oral suspension, but they need different doses. After evaluating the families' situation, the pharmacist might decide that the best strategy for compliance for all 3 children would be to dilute the medication to 3 mg/mL. This will provide the mother with an easy way to measure the different dose for each child (ie, 3 mg/1 mL for the smallest child, 6 mg/2 mL for the next child, and 9 mg/3 mL for the largest child). The pharmacy would write an MFR to dilute the commercial Tamiflu (6 mg/mL) to the new concentration of 3 mg/mL. The dispensing label must also reflect the new concentration. This is now a compounded medication. Professional judgment was used to evaluate and find the easiest way for this mom to accurately deliver the doses. Calculation was performed to determine the accurate dilution to make dosing easy and accurate. The label placed on the medication reflects the dose concentration that is *dispensed* rather than the dose concentration of the manufactured product.

Diluting a manufactured medication to reduce the strength *is* compounding.
Reconstitution of a manufactured product is *not* compounding.

ORAL LIQUIDS

When a patient cannot swallow a tablet or capsule, or when a manufactured liquid dosage form is unsuitable for the patient's drug therapy, a compounded oral liquid is often prescribed. Compounding an oral liquid can be as simple as adding a flavor to a reconstituted antibiotic or as complex as putting several drugs in proper amounts into one preparation. In all of these, the technician's skill and knowledge is crucial to the patient receiving the proper medication.

There are 5 common types of vehicles used in the preparation of compounded oral liquid medications (Table 5-1). A vehicle is an **inert** medium in which an active drug is administered.

TABLE 5-1 Common Vehicles for Compounding Oral Liquids

Vehicle	
Water	Used for drugs soluble in water Short BUD
Oil	Used for drugs soluble in oil Extends the medication's BUD
Syrups	Combination of water and sweetener
Structured suspending vehicles	Contains excipient ingredients to thicken water
Elixirs	Sweetened liquid containing alcohol

Water

Water contains no sugar, no carbohydrates or calories, and no preservatives, dyes, or fragrances. It also contains no gluten, corn, or other common dietary allergens. Water might be the only appropriate vehicle for some patients who must avoid these materials. However, water is the most effective growth media for all living things, including microorganisms and bacteria that are harmful to humans. This means that within 10 to 15 days, an unwanted microorganism or bacteria in water will grow and multiply.

Purified water is the type of water listed most often in MFR for compounded oral liquids. Purified water is also called **distilled water**. Water is distilled by boiling it to remove impurities. The steam from the boiling water is then captured and put into a clean container.

Preserved water is purified water with preservatives added to it. The preservatives prevent microbes that might have entered the water in the compounding process from growing. Preserved water contains the common preservatives methyl paraben and propyl paraben. The technician must be careful to use preserved water only when it is written into the MFR. If preserved water is used in place of purified water in a medication made for a patient who has allergies to these types of preservatives, the medication would cause them harm.

Adding water to any product shortens the stability. The stability of compounded liquid containing water is based primarily on how long the active pharmaceutical ingredient (API) can be in the presence of water before it degrades. However, an equally important factor is how long the vehicle can be expected to avoid microbial growth. Most vehicles contain preservatives so that microbes will not grow during the course of therapy. Think back to the azithromycin example discussed earlier. The powders in the manufactured product have an expiration date. This date is often quite long—years in fact. However, the BUD of the oral suspension (once the water is added) is usually between 7 and 14 days. Aqueous preparations often require refrigeration after mixing to maintain their stability and potency.

Oils

The oils used as vehicles for liquid compounded dosage forms are called **fixed oils**. These pharmaceutical grade liquids are generally the oil squeezed from a plant. "Fixed" means that the oil cannot burn without external ignition (fire) and that they do not evaporate. The primary benefit of using oil as the vehicle for an oral liquid is that the chance of harmful organisms growing in the preparation is reduced. In general, oils do not support microbial growth. Per USP/NF Chapter <795> monograph, compounded liquids in oil vehicles can be assigned a BUD of 6 months from the date they were prepared. This is much longer than the BUD allowed for compounded liquids prepared in aqueous vehicles. Because some drugs that are well absorbed through mucous membranes are also **soluble** in fixed oils, oil is frequently used as a vehicle in the preparation of oral medications delivered as sublingual drops. If a drug that is not soluble in oil is compounded into an oil vehicle, the drug will be in suspension. Using an oil vehicle for these drugs is not suggested because it is difficult to shake well, causing inaccuracy in dosing.

Syrups

Syrup is sweetened water. Syrup is very palatable and the taste of many drugs can be improved by its sweetness. Simple syrup USP is a specific combination of water and sugar in approximately a 1:1 proportion. Simple syrup USP has no flavor or preservatives and is only stable for 14 days refrigerated. Therefore, until recently compounding pharmacies would need to prepare it quite often. Most pharmacies now purchase manufactured syrups that include preservatives and have expirations dates much longer than 14 days. These manufactured syrups are made from sucrose USP (the chemical name for sugar) and water in the same proportions as simple syrup USP, but with pharmaceutical grade preservatives added. Manufactured flavored syrups (cherry, grape, orange, bubblegum, raspberry, etc) are also available and frequently used in compounded medications. Manufacturers who provide compounding vehicles also provide sugar-free syrups that use nonreducing sugars to sweeten water.

Sorbitol 70% solution is syrup made from nonreducing sugars. It is frequently used in liquid formulations that must be sugar free.

Glycerin is a slightly sweet, thick substance that is often added to sorbitol 70% solution to add suspension properties to the oral liquid being prepared.

Structured Suspending Vehicles

A **structured suspending vehicle** is an aqueous vehicle that has been formulated to provide adequate suspension of particles in a compounded oral liquid. In simple terms, it is stable, thickened water. It is not very palatable, but drugs that are soluble in water dissolve in it when a sugar-free solution is required, and drugs with no water solubility can be suspended and reshaken to provide even distribution of powder particles in a compounded suspension.

Methylcellulose gel is water that has been thickened with methylcellulose to create a better suspending vehicle. Methylcellulose gel is the simplest of structured suspending vehicles. Methylcellulose is a pharmaceutical grade of the cellulose material used to make paper or cardboard. When water is added to methylcellulose powder, the powder floats to the top. A whisk or stir-rod is used to disturb this mass of powder to expose the particles to the water. The powder soaks up the water and becomes a gelatinous mass floating on the water. With stirring, the mass dissolves into the water and the finished product is thick enough to suspend powders but thin enough to pour. In the vast majority of pharmacies, compounded methylcellulose gel has been replaced by commercial structured suspending vehicles. For example, Ora-Plus is a commonly used manufactured methylcellulose gel. These commercial products contain preservatives.

In traditional compounding, a 1:1 *combination* of syrup and methylcellulose gel was the most common vehicle used to provide oral liquids. In modern compounding, these 2 most basic liquids are used only in special cases in which they are the best way to provide an oral liquid suitable for a patient who cannot tolerate preservatives. Modern pharmacies generally utilize the manufactured syrups (ie, bubble gum syrup) and structured suspending vehicles (ie, methylcellulose gel 2%) in some combination instead. The most common combination is a 1:1 mixture of an oral suspending vehicle and an oral syrup vehicle. These two products can be measured and mixed together in whatever proportion is best for a particular compound. There are also "one-step" suspending systems that combine the suspending and sweetening vehicles into one product.

Other "one-step" vehicles are available, which use **starch NF** rather than methylcellulose as the suspending agent. The starch-based system (the water is thickened with starch instead of methylcellulose) seems to keep powders in suspension for a longer time, and patients do not suffer the gastrointestinal (GI) distress (diarrhea) that is commonly associated with long-term use of methylcellulose or sorbitol-based vehicles.

Elixirs

An **elixir** is an oral liquid medication that contains at least 10% alcohol. Because alcohol is a drug itself and one that is regulated by more federal agencies than the Food and Drug Administration (FDA), prescriptions for elixirs are rare. In an elixir, alcohol is used to

Always **question the use of alcohol preparations for children, patients with substance abuse history, or patients taking other medications that may interact with alcohol.**

completely dissolve the drug. A syrup or structured vehicle is then added to the drug solution to complete the volume. Adding a few drops of alcohol to increase powder solubility and then adding an aqueous vehicle to create a final volume is not an elixir. A technician should question the use of alcohol in patients with a history of substance abuse, or patients taking other medications that may interact with alcohol, in order to avoid harm to the patient. *Children should not be given elixirs* unless instructed by a physician.

FLAVORING FOR ORAL LIQUIDS

Flavoring of an oral liquid is the addition of a substance to the medication that was not present in the commercially manufactured product. *Adding flavoring, even to a reconstituted medication is considered compounding*, and should be labeled appropriately. The BUD is seldom changed by the addition of a flavor, but a reference is needed to either prove this or to document the professional judgment used to assign a new BUD.

A wide variety of water-**miscible** flavors, which are used in water-based vehicles, and oil-miscible flavors, which are added to oil vehicles, are available. It is important to choose the correct type of liquid flavor. Water-miscible flavors are normally artificial or natural flavors in a **propylene glycol** solution. Propylene glycol is a common solvent that is safe for consumption in small amounts. Oil-miscible flavors are often essential oils extracted from the roots, leaves, and fruits of various plants. Powder flavors can be used in either water or oil vehicles.

In general, flavoring agents are considered safe and do not alter the stability of the preparation. Flavoring manufacturers often provide suggested guidelines for how much flavoring is needed based on the drug, the liquid vehicle, and/or the volume being prepared. Some compounding pharmacies may choose to standardize the amount of flavoring they add to compounded oral liquids. For example, a pharmacy may have a standard procedure of adding flavors at 0.5% of the total volume of the preparation. This amount is calculated and applied to every MFR for a compounded oral liquid. However, flavors are intended to improve compliance, so flavoring agents should be "tweeked" to make the medication pleasing to the patients' taste. A useful flavoring strategy is to combine different flavors. For example, if a patient complains that an oral liquid still tastes bad after the addition of cherry flavoring, adding of a few drops of chocolate flavoring might solve the problem.

Most flavoring agents are alcohol-free, dye-free, and sugar-free and safe for patients with allergies to specific food dyes, etc. Liquid flavors generally have short expiration dating.

Adding flavoring to a medication *is* considered compounding.

In addition to flavoring agents, **bitterness maskers** are also available in both liquid or powder forms. These products are usually sugar-free combinations of nonreducing sugars (those that do not add calories) and/or **stevia**. These are often an option for patients that need to avoid added sugars. Just remember that adding more sweetness to a preparation does not always make it more palatable.

LIQUIDS ADMINISTERED BY TUBE FEEDING

Many patients receive their medications through tubes that deliver food and medication directly into the stomach. **NG-tubes (nasogastric tubes)** enter the stomach through the nose. **G-tubes (gastronomy tube)** enter the stomach through a port surgically placed in the abdomen.

Water-soluble drugs delivered through tubes often use water alone as the vehicle. Because water is thin, it is less likely to clog the tube compared to a structured vehicle. This makes administration easier and less time consuming for the caregiver, especially a nonprofessional, such as a family member. Water can also be used alone as the vehicle for a drug without water solubility. A water suspension must be shaken vigorously as all the drug will settle out of the liquid between administrations. Methylcellulose gel may be a better vehicle for tube administration. The thickened water will suspend the drug better than plain water, ensuring delivery of a more accurate dose in each administration. It is less likely to clog the tube. Sweetness and flavor are not necessary in the case of tube administration.

SUBLINGUAL LIQUIDS

Sublingual drops are delivered under the tongue and absorbed rapidly through the mucous membrane. A compounded sublingual drop is often an excellent method of delivering tiny amounts of oil-soluble drugs that can be absorbed from the tissue under the tongue. Oral vitamins and sometimes hormones are delivered sublingually in a compounded liquid. For example, a 2 mg dose of estrogen can be delivered in as little as 0.1 mL of a fixed oil. The drug is dissolved in the oil and an oil miscible flavor, and perhaps a powdered sweetening agent is added. The preparation is dispensed in a small bottle with an oral syringe. The patient withdraws 0.1 mL of the oily solution from the container using the marks on the syringe to measure accurately. This tiny amount of liquid contains 1 dose that is held under the tongue until it has been completely absorbed. It is important that the patient is educated on the use of the medication, so that neither the sublingual drop nor the saliva under the tongue is swallowed. Although the name implies using a dropper bottle to dispense sublingual drops, an oral syringe should always be used to ensure accurate dosing (Table 5-2).

TABLE 5-2 Example Master Formula Record for Sublingual Drops

Master Formula Record: Testosterone 10 mg/0.1 mL Sublingual Drops to Make 3 mL	
Supplies and Equipment 2—10 cc Luer-Lock syringes (see Chapter 7) 1—luer to luer connector (see Chapter 7) 1—1 oz amber container with childproof cap 1—press-in adapter compatible with bottle opening 3—1 mL oral amber syringes with caps	
Ingredients	**Amounts Needed**
Testosterone micronized USP	0.3 g
Peppermint flavoring (OM)	0.1 mL
Stevia NF	0.1 g
Grape seed oil NF **(QS AD)**	3.0 mL
Procedures	
1. Accurately weigh and measure testosterone USP, peppermint flavoring (OM), and stevia.	
2. Remove plunger from one 10 cc luer lock syringe and connect it to the other 10 cc luer lock syringe with the LL to LL connector. Align the connected syringes vertically with the open LL syringe on top.	
3. Place testosterone USP powder in the open luer lock syringe.	
4. Add stevia and flavoring to the open luer lock syringe.	
5. Add grape seed oil to the open luer lock syringe until volume of 3 cc is reached.	
6. Replace plunger into the open luer lock syringe, just to break the seal.	
7. Flip the connected syringes so that the top is on the bottom.	
8. Remove the connector and top syringe from the bottom syringe.	
9. Gently press the plunger in the syringe containing the preparation to remove any air.	
10. Reconnect the syringes and press the material from one syringe to the other to thoroughly mix the ingredients and dissolve the powders.	
11. Press all the material into one luer lock syringe and remove the connector and the empty syringe.	
12. Press all the material from the luer lock syringe into a 1 oz amber container with childproof closure.	
13. Insert press-in adaptor in the neck of the bottle. Apply childproof closure.	
14. Label: Deliver 0.1 mL under tongue once daily for thirty days.	
15. Dispense with oral syringe labeled with 0.1 mL scale.	

Magic Mouthwash

A very common compounded liquid is known as **"magic mouthwash"** (MMW). Although magic mouthwash is usually a **swish and spit** preparation that would technically qualify it as a topical liquid, it will be discussed with the other liquids that are delivered orally as it may be swallowed, either accidentally or per the prescriber's instruction. Magic mouthwashes are used to treat pain caused by mucositis from chemo and radiation therapies and mouth ulcers (aphthous ulcers). The liquid is swished around inside the mouth for a certain amount of time then spitting it out.

Magic mouthwash often contains an anti-infective, a steroid to strengthen the tissue and decrease inflammation and an anesthetic to soothe pain. It may also include a coating agent (often an antacid), and/or an antihistamine. There are dozens of formulations for MMW. Most institutional and compounding pharmacies will prepare it on a regular basis. Even a pharmacy that does very little compounding will have some variation of magic mouthwash available to patients with a prescription. Most are simple combinations of 2 or more manufactured liquids (Tables 5-3 and 5-4).

TABLE 5-3 Sample of Magic Mouthwash Formulation

Magic Mouthwash Total Volume 200 mL	
Nystatin suspension	40 mL
Dexamethasone 4 mg/mL	0.56 mL
Distilled water	QS to 200 mL
Directions: Swish and spit 5 mL QID.	

TABLE 5-4 Sample of Magic Mouthwash Formulation

Magic Mouthwash Gargle Solution	
2% viscous lidocaine	30 mL
Diphenhydramine 2.5 mg/mL	30 mL
Maalox	60 mL
Carafate 1 g/10 mL	40 mL
Directions: Swish, gargle, and spit 5-10 mL Q6H AD.	

TOPICAL LIQUIDS

As discussed in Chapter 1, a compounded medication can be used to treat a condition that requires a strength or concentration that is not commercially available, or a combination of products that may be used to effectively treat multiple symptoms of a particular patient. This is the reason for the compounding of many topical liquid preparations. For example, perhaps a patient needs a strong combination of a steroid and an anesthetic to soothe the discomfort caused by a bug bite or exposure to a toxic plant. Often, the prescribed drugs are available commercially only as creams or ointments. If the condition of the patient is so severe that touching the area is torturous, the physician might prescribe a compounded topical solution of the drug or drugs that can be applied through a spray. The compounded topical liquid represents a change in dosage form, and also the best treatment option for this patient.

Caustic materials are regularly used to treat fungal infections. Because these chemicals are hazardous, manufactured products are often supplied in doses that are not effective in treating resistant strains of a particular **fungus**. If the prescriber determines that a more potent dose or a combination therapy is required, a compounded topical liquid may be the best treatment option. Compounded topical solutions frequently utilize drugs with no water solubility so alcohol is a common vehicle for such preparations.

It is important to use caution when handling caustic materials. Technicians should wear gloves and other PPE when preparing products that include hazardous drug ingredients.

ENEMAS AND DOUCHES

In a compounding pharmacy practice, you may also prepare enemas and douches. These dosage forms normally use an aqueous vehicle and contain water-soluble materials. An enema is a liquid that is administered to the rectum. A douche is a liquid used to deliver medication to the vagina.

Enema

The purpose of enema therapy is to cause the bowel to contract and stimulate the normal excretion process to completely void the bowel of any stool inside it. Enema is also the name commonly used to refer to the liquid that is introduced into the rectum and/or colon via the anus to achieve this result. Enemas are sometimes prescribed in cases when natural peristalsis is compromised for some reason causing severe and dangerous constipation. Enema liquids are compounded most frequently in an institutional setting to clear the rectum in preparation for a GI procedure. The enema is necessary to remove any waste that could cause infection and/or other complications. Compounded enemas are normally given on an as needed basis and are only prepared with a physician's order for one, scheduled administration. The enema is prepared just before administration, so beyond-use dating (BUD) is not applicable. Institutions use a variety of simple formulations; many of them do not contain any active drug ingredients (Table 5-5).

TABLE 5-5 Sample of Compounded Enema Formulation

Milk and Molasses Enema—for Severe Constipation	
Supplies and equipment **Enema bag** **Lubricant**	
Warm-hot tap water	180 mL
Powdered milk (do not use cow's milk)	90 mL
Molasses	135 mL
Instructions	
1. Mix water and powdered milk in a container.	
2. Add the molasses. Stir again until the mixture has an even color.	
3. Pour the milk and molasses mixture into the enema bag.	
4. Remove air from the tube by opening the clamp and allowing the mixture to completely fill the tube. Raise the end of the tube higher than the bag and lower it gradually to avoid leakage.	
5. Close tube clamp.	
6. Administer to patient as per institutional protocol and procedures.	

Douches

Douche therapy is the introduction of water into the vagina to rinse or deliver medication to the vaginal cavity. Douches are often prepared and administered in an institutional setting, but are also dispensed to be administered at home. A douche is administered (or self-administered) while the patient is on the toilet or in the shower and the drugs mixed with liquid simply flows in to the vagina and back out. Active drugs are more common in douches than in enemas. They are an excellent way to deliver an antifungal medication, an anesthetic drug, like lidocaine, or a fortified dose of an antibiotic.

SOURCE OF DRUG

There are 2 primary sources of the medication used in compounded liquids: **MDF** (manufactured drug formulations) and active pharmaceutical ingredients (APIs). Most often, a compounded oral liquid is ordered simply to deliver the proper medication to a patient who cannot swallow a tablet or capsule. If this can be accomplished successfully by crushing the tablet and suspending the powder in the correct vehicle, the manufactured drug should be used. If a very accurate dose and volume is required, for example in a topical solution, it may be best to use the purest form, an API powder.

For an API to be used legitimately in a compounded liquid one of two justifications must be involved:

- No suitable manufactured formulation of the drug is available.
- There is a patient-specific reason that the commercial product that is available is not suitable as the source-of-drug.

The source of drug has an important effect on the master formulation record (MFR). For example, to provide 250 mg/mL of a drug from the API in 100 mL of an oral compounded liquid, you will simply weigh 25 g of the powder. When the same 100 mL of 250 mg/mL liquid is prepared from crushed 250 mg tablets, the powder used will weigh *more* than 25 g because it will include the excipient ingredients contained in the tablets. The excipients contribute weight and they also take up more space in the final product. Giving the instruction *QS AD* in the amount column in the MFR gives a direction that will work for either the 25 g of API or the larger amount of powder derived from the crushed tablets. Regardless of the amount of powder you put into the conical cylinder, adding the vehicle to the powder with geometric dilution always yields the proper amount of medication (the proper dose per mL). Resulting in a accurate medication customized to meet the needs of a specific patient. Remember that skipping the step of levigation before addition of the vehicle tends to make the powders clump together resulting in uneven dosing.

BEYOND-USE DATING

As discussed in Chapter 4, each compounded medication must be assigned a beyond-use date (BUD) and the pharmacist must be able to document a reference for BUD of the compounded drug. As discussed earlier in this chapter, microorganisms can flourish in water. The USP/NF Chapter <795> monograph provides default BUD standards for aqueous liquids when no documented stability information is available. A compounded oral liquid (to be swallowed) containing water must be assigned a BUD of *14 days* from the date prepared. The standard BUD established in USP/NF Chapter <795> for a compounded liquid in an oil vehicle is *6 months*. However, there are very little published data available on drugs in oils. In other words, oils should not replace aqueous vehicles just to achieve a longer BUD (see Chapter 4, Table 4-2).

Special Considerations and Extended Dating

Some drugs have special considerations that can affect their stability in compounded *oral* liquid preparations. Stability of a suspension or solution is often affected by the pH (measurement of acidity) of the preparation. For example, proton pump inhibitors (ie, omeprazole and lansoprazole) compounded into suspensions must have a pH greater than 7.8 to prevent the acidic environment of the stomach from destroying their potency. In these cases, extended BUD can only be applied if the vehicle provides a stable **alkaline** pH throughout the course of therapy.

Two other drugs that must be given special considerations are *aspirin* and *nystatin*; *aspirin* begins to degrade in the presence of water within about 2 hours, so it should never be mixed in an aqueous vehicle. There are published formulations for aspirin in nonaqueous vehicles and these preparations may be labeled with a 3-month BUD per USP/NF Chapter <795>.

Nystatin should not be compounded as an aqueous, sugar-free suspension. Nystatin suspension is commercially available as an aqueous oral liquid *containing sugar*. The syrup protects the nystatin from degradation in this preparation. In the presence of water, and without the sugar, nystatin begins to degrade almost immediately. Contact the manufacturer of the nystatin for information about how nystatin can be delivered orally for a patient that cannot have sugar.

Documentation of extended dating benefits both the pharmacy preparing medication and the patient. *The Stability of Compounded Preparations* by Lawrence Trissel has been a valuable resource for documenting extended BUDs for many years. The drug monographs in this reference provide the abstracts of studies performed by **high-performance liquid chromatography (HPLC)** on many active drugs in various vehicles. HPLC testing is used to document the concentration of active drug in the specific preparation studied. HPLC testing is performed at certain time increments and under certain storage conditions and the results document what is commonly referred to as **stability** of the drug.

The BUD documented by HPLC applies *only* to the preparation studied. However, because most suspending vehicles are basically equivalent, the pharmacist often uses professional judgment to assign an equivalent BUD to a preparation made with an alternative but equivalent vehicle. Many manufacturers of compounding vehicles invest in HPLC testing of select drugs prepared using their products to document acceptable extended BUDs. If these data are available, they will be available on the vehicle manufacturer's website.

STORAGE CONDITIONS

Specific storage conditions of a compounded liquid must appear on the dispensing label. These may include refrigeration, protect from light, etc. Storage conditions are critical to the stability of many compounded preparations and will be listed in the labeling section of the MFR. Storage conditions are also critical to the stability of manufactured drug formulations, active pharmaceutical ingredients, and manufactured compounding vehicles. Table 5-6 lists USP/NF storage requirements guidelines and temperature ranges used for both compounded and commercially manufactured products.

TABLE 5-6 Temperature and Storage Guidelines

Storage and Temperature Conditions	USP Definition
Freezer	Temperature maintained at between −25° and −10°C
Refrigerator	Temperature maintained between 2° and 8°C
Cold	Any temperature not exceeding 8°C
Cool	Temperatures between 8° and 15°C
Room temperature	General temperature prevailing in a work environment
Controlled room temperature	Temperatures between 20° and 25°C
	Excursions are allowed between 15° and 30°C in pharmacies, hospitals, and warehouses
	Spikes up to 40°C are permitted for no more than 24 h
Warm	Temperature ranges between 30° and 40°C
Excessive heat	Any temperature between 30° and 40°C
Dry place	Does not exceed 40% humidity at 20°C
Protection from freezing	Freezing will cause a loss of potency or strength or a destructive alteration of properties to the product
Protection from light	Light will cause a loss of strength or potency or a destructive alteration of properties to the product

INSTRUCTIONS FOR USE

While manufactured medications must provide a package insert that contains detailed information about the medication for use by both the pharmacist and the patient, compounded medications do not require this document.

Instead the primary dispensing label must include the following:

- The name of the formulation
- The dose and administration directions, also known as the "Sig"
- The route of administration, for example "by mouth" or "under the tongue"

- Storage conditions and warnings that apply to the medication
- A BUD
- Auxiliary labels

CONCLUSION

In a compounding facility, it is a common practice to prepare liquids for patients for whom an manufactured formulation is not appropriate. The technician who prepares compounded liquid medications should have the knowledge and skills necessary to properly combine powders and liquid vehicles, to calculate changes in drug concentration by dilution or allegation, and to assist in identifying the best way to dispense liquids based on patient needs.

CHAPTER SUMMARY

- Non-sterile (NS) liquid dosage forms can be delivered orally, directly into the stomach, to the skin or into the rectum or vagina.
- Liquid dosage forms delivered to the eye, nose, bloodstream, or respiratory system are sterile compounds and cannot be prepared in an NS setting.
- A solution is a mixture of liquid and powder in which the powder is completely dissolved in the liquid.
- A suspension is a mixture of liquid and powder in which the powder is surrounded by the liquid.
- Reconstitution is not compounding.
- Adding more water than is recommended by the manufacturer is dilution.
- Dilution of a manufactured oral liquid is compounding.
- The 5 most common oral liquid vehicles include the following:
  Water
  Oil
  Suspending vehicles
  Syrups
  Elixirs
- Water is an effective growth media for living things.
- Preserved water contains methyl paraben and propyl paraben.
- Adding water to anything may shorten its stability.
- Oil does not promote the growth of harmful bacteria.
- Methylcellulose gel is thickened water.
- Syrup is sweetened water.
- Glycerin is a slightly sweet, thick substance that is often added to sorbitol 70% solution to add suspension properties to a compounded oral liquid.
- Starch is a desirable suspending agent because:
  Drugs remain in suspension for a longer time.
  It does not cause GI distress or diarrhea.
- An elixir is a liquid medication that contains at least 10% alcohol.
- Alcohol is usually avoided in compounded formulations for children and the elderly.
- Sublingual drops are delivered under the tongue and the medication is absorbed through the mucous membrane.
- Magic mouthwash (MMW) is used to treat pain caused by mucositis from chemo and radiation therapies and mouth ulcers.
- An enema is a liquid that is administered to the rectum.

- Many enema formulations do not contain any active drug ingredients.
- A douche is a liquid used to deliver medication to the vagina.
- The two primary sources of the medication used in compounded liquids include the following:
  Prepared dosage forms
  Active pharmaceutical ingredients (APIs).
- Oils should not replace liquids just to achieve a longer BUD.
- Specific storage conditions of a compounded liquid must appear on the dispensing label.
- Auxiliary labels must never cover the information on the primary label.

PTCB Review Questions

1. What is the standard BUD for oral liquids in an aqueous medium per the USP/NF Chapter <795> monograph on NS compounding?
   A. 3 months
   B. 10 days
   C. 14 days
   D. 6 weeks
2. Which products are often compounded for sublingual administration?
   A. Anti-infective agents
   B. Vitamins
   C. Hormones
   D. Both B and C
3. From what sources are "fixed oils" derived?
   A. Plants
   B. Plants and animal products
   C. Animal fats
   D. Water
4. What ingredient is required for a compounded oral liquid to be considered an elixir?
   A. Water
   B. Oil
   C. Alcohol
   D. Starch
5. What percentage of alcohol is needed to prepare an elixir?
   A. At least 20%
   B. At least 10%
   C. 0%
   D. At least 5%
6. Identify the *true* statement regarding compounding liquid formulations.
   A. Many enema formulations do not contain any active drug ingredients.
   B. An enema is administered through an NG tube.
   C. An enema is a liquid that is administered to the rectum.
   D. A and C are true statements.
7. Which is the USP/NF default BUD for liquid compounded products that use oil as the vehicle?
   A. 14 days
   B. 6 months
   C. 60 days
   D. 4 weeks
8. Which of the following is a *false* statement?
   A. Adding a flavoring agent is not considered compounding.
   B. Reconstitution of a commercial product is considered compounding.
   C. Both A and B.
   D. Dilution of a manufactured product is considered compounding.

9. What ingredient is commonly added to create preserved water?
   A. Methylcellulose gel
   B. Methyl paraben
   C. Sorbitol
   D. Glycerin
10. What product should not be prepared in an aqueous vehicle?
    A. Aspirin
    B. Syrup
    C. Suspension
    D. MMW

Techs in Practice: Discussion Topics and Questions

SCENARIO 1

Use the Internet to find 3 common agents used in compounded topical liquid **wart** preparations.

1. Find a material safety data sheet (MSDS) on each agent and list the precautions that need to be taken when preparing compounds using these APIs.
2. Are any of these agents used in commercially available wart preparations?
3. What auxiliary labels should be added to the dispensing label?

SCENARIO 2

Cantharidin USP is a powerful caustic agent that dissolves severe types of warts. A cantharidin solution is always in acetone or alcohol and contains no water. This caustic medication is provided in 0.7% concentration and only a small amount of the preparation is dispensed. It is applied with a dropper, directly to the wart. A manufacture provides this drug in premeasured **aliquots** of API powder that is used to create a 10 mL total volume.

How would you package this product for dispensing?

What BUD would you give this product?

What PPE is required when preparing this drug?

Are there specific instructions and/or equipment the patient will need to administer and store this product correctly?

What are the advantages of the individual aliquot packages?

Lab 1

A prescription for oral nystatin will be written to provide a certain number of "international units" (IUs). In order to provide a patient with the correct dose of nystatin without any sugar, the pharmacy will dispense nystatin as the API powder. The "activity" of the API is given as the number of international units (IUs) per milligram. Each lot of nystatin has a specific activity that is printed on the label and on the certificate of analysis (C of A). The nystatin powder is dispensed, in an amount sufficient to complete the course of therapy.

The patient uses the calibrated measuring spoon or scoops to remove the powder needed for a dose and adds the powder to a food or beverage at time of administration.

A prescription is received for *14,400 IUs/dose of nystatin sugar-free. Dispense 10 doses.* Nystatin is not stable in a sugar-free liquid vehicle and must be dispensed as powder to be added to food or beverage at time of administration.
The C of A for the nystatin USP powder in stock has an activity of 5485 IU/mg.

1. Calculate the number of milligrams of powder needed to supply 1 dose.
2. Calculate the number of milligrams of powder needed to supply the full 10 doses.
3. How would the pharmacy staff determine what spoon or scoop would be appropriate to dispense with the powder?

Lab 2

Use the Internet or other sources to find *MMW* recipes.

1. Find two formulations that contain an antacid and an antihistamine.
2. Find one formulation that contains an antibiotic and a corticosteroid or anti-inflammatory.
3. Find two formulations that contain an anesthetic.
4. Find one formulation that contains all the ingredients listed previously.

Calculation Review Questions

A prescription is presented for a compounded medication: *Metronidazole 250 mg/5 mL SF oral liquid; dispense 90 mL.*

1. Calculate the number of metronidazole 250 mg tablets needed to prepare this medication.
2. Calculate the number of metronidazole 500 mg tablets needed to prepare this medication.

The compounding pharmacy knows that compliance is greater in patients who receive metronidazole as a compounded oral liquid prepared using metronidazole benzoate USP active pharmaceutical ingredient powder.
1.6 g of metronidazole benzoate is equivalent to 1 g of metronidazole.

3. Calculate the amount of metronidazole benzoate powder that must be weighed/measured to prepare this compounded oral liquid.

The pharmacy has received a prescription for 1000 mL (liter) of a simple 3% acetic acid douche. The acetic acid available in the pharmacy stock is acetic acid 5% solution.

4. Calculate the correct amount of acetic acid 5% solution needed to prepare compounded liquid preparation.

This chapter includes the following PTCE Blueprint Knowledge Areas
Section 1.0-1.4 Strengths/dose, dosage forms, physical appearance, routes of administration, and duration of drug therapy.
Section 2.0-2.6 Record keeping, documentation, and retention (eg, length of time prescriptions are maintained on file).
Section 2.0-2.11 Infection control standards (eg, laminar air flow, clean room, hand washing, cleaning counting trays, countertop, and equipment) (OSHA, USP/NF Chapter ⟨795⟩ and ⟨797⟩).
Section 2.0-2.13 Professional standards regarding the roles and responsibilities of pharmacist, pharmacy technicians, and other pharmacy employees. (TJC, BOP)
Section 2.0-2.15 Facility, equipment, and supply requirements (eg, space requirements, prescription file storage, cleanliness, reference materials). (TJC, USP, BOP)
Section 3.0-3.3 Documentation (eg, batch preparation, compounding record).
Section 3.0-3.5 Selection and use of equipment and supplies.
Section 3.0-3.7 Non-sterile compounding processes.
Section 6.0-6.3 Calculate dosing required.
Section 6.0-6.4 Fill process (eg, select appropriate product, apply special handling requirements, measure and prepare product for final check).
Section 6.0-6.5 Labeling requirements (eg, auxiliary and warning labels, expiration date, patient specific information).
Section 6.0 Packaging requirements (eg, types of bags, syringes, glass, PVC, child resistant, light resistant).

This chapter includes the following Ex-CPT Test Specifications

Section 1 A-4 Comply with rules and regulations when filling prescriptions.

Section 1 A-6 Maintain a clean work environment in the pharmacy and patient care areas.

Section 1 C-7 Properly package prescription medication in child-resistant containers or other approved containers as required.

Section 1 C-8 Comply with professional, state, and federal laws and regulations.

Section 1 C-9 Use information found on medication stock bottles, such as drug name and strength, expiration date, and lot number.

Section 2 A-2 Differentiate among various dosage forms (eg, tablets vs capsules, ointment vs creams, controlled release vs immediate release, parenteral vs oral).

Section 3 B-2 Identify drugs that require special handling procedures.

Section 3 B-5 Follow proper record keeping procedures pertaining to the pharmacy.

Section 3 B-6 Follow the pharmacy's quality assurance policies and procedures.

Section 3 B-14 Properly and accurately prepare prescription labels.

Section 3 B-18 Use auxiliary labels properly.

Section 3 B-19 Properly label drug products packaged in approved containers or, when appropriate, original packages.

Section 3 C-2 Calculate the quantities of prescription medications to be dispensed.

Section 3 C-4 Properly calculate individual and daily dosages.

Section 3 D-1 Follow proper compounding procedures for NS products.

Section 3 D-3 Properly repackage and label unit of use products.

Section 3 D-4 Properly calculate expiration dates for repackaged products.

This chapter includes the following ASHP Model Curriculum for Pharmacy Technician Training Goal Statements, Objectives, and Instructional Objectives

OBJ 2.4 Efficiently secure information to complete a prescription/medication order.

OBJ 3.3 Follow established laws and protocols to select the appropriate product.

OBJ 3.5 Accurately count or measure finished dosage forms as specified by the prescription/medication order.

OBJ 3.6 Collect the correct ingredients for sterile or NS products that require compounding.

OBJ 3.7 Accurately determine the correct amounts of ingredients for a compounded product.

OBJ 3.11 Follow safety policies and procedures in the preparation of all medications.

OBJ 3.13 Package the product in the appropriate type and size of container using a manual process or automated system.

OBJ 3.14 Follow an established manual procedure or electronic procedure to generate accurate and complete product labels.

OBJ 3.18 Follow established policies and procedures for recording the preparation of bulk, unit dose, and special doses of medications prepared for immediate or in anticipation of future use.

OBJ 3.19 Follow the manufacturer's recommendation and/or the pharmacy's guidelines for storage of all medications prior to distribution.

Answers to PTCB Review Questions

1. **C**
2. **D**
3. **A**
4. **C**
5. **B**
6. **D**
7. **B**
8. **C**
9. **B**
10. **A**

Answers to Calculation Questions

1. 18
2. 9
3. 7.2 g
4. 600 mL

CHAPTER

6 Solid Dosage Forms

INTRODUCTION

Solid dosage forms offer the ability to combine several drugs into one product helping increase patient compliance and in many cases, improving product stability. Solid dosage forms can provide an opportunity to meet the need of a particular patient, delivered in a convenient manner. This chapter explains the various compounded solid dosage forms available and discuss techniques and tools that streamline and enhance the compounding process.

LEARNING OBJECTIVES

- Describe the different types of solid dosage forms and explain the purpose of each.
- Describe the supplies and equipment needed to prepare solid dosage forms.
- Discuss the different ingredients used in preparing solid dosage forms.
- Describe the process for capsule filling.
- Explain the process for preparing rapid dissolving tablets (RDTs) and tablet triturates (TTs).
- Describe the process for preparing medicinal troches and lollipops and lip balms.
- Explain the process for preparing suppositories.
- Explain the importance of quality assurance measures for solid dosage forms.
- Explain the parameters for beyond use dating for each solid dosage form.

KEY TERMS

Cavity: A hollowed out area in an object

Cellulose: Pharmaceutical grade product derived from plant materials used as an excipient in capsules

Gelatin: Pharmaceutical grade product derived from cattle, fish, or pork, used as the main ingredient in capsule shells

Overencapsulation: Placing a commercially available tablet into a capsule shell

PEG: Polyethylene glycol, a synthetic wax produced in various molecular weights

"Punch" method: A traditional hand filling procedure for filling capsules containing active pharmaceutical ingredients (APIs) and excipients

Tamper: A tool used to press powders into the base of a capsule, when using a precision capsule machine

Veggie caps: Capsules formed from cellulose

CAPSULES

A compounded capsule can be the best choice for patients for the following reasons:

- The correct dose is not available in a manufactured product.
- The manufactured version of a drug contains additives that can cause an adverse reaction in the patient.
- Delivery of multiple drugs in one capsule may improve compliance for a patient having difficulty swallowing multiple tablets of a prescribed medication.

Capsules are most frequently used to deliver medication to the stomach and small intestine for absorption through the gastrointestinal (GI) tract. They can also provide a simple container or vehicle for the correct dose of a medication to be administered.

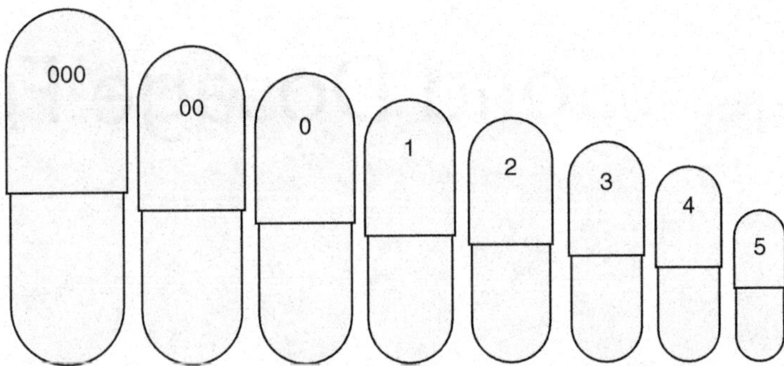

FIGURE 6-1 Capsule sizes.

The proper dose of a drug can be measured by the pharmacy and placed inside a capsule. It can then be opened and the contents sprinkled on top of food or added to a beverage at time of administration. This strategy is often used to increase the stability and shelf life of a medication and for ease of administration to elderly patients or children. Additionally, a capsule can be delivered intravaginally as a suppository.

Capsules are composed of either **gelatin** or **cellulose**, and the manufacturing process is the same for both types. The gelatin used to form capsule shells is a pharmaceutical grade of the gelatin obtained from cattle, fish, or pork. Cellulose capsules are derived from a pharmaceutical grade plant material and are commonly referred to as "veggie caps." **Veggie caps** are frequently used in patients that have dietary restrictions that include animal protein.

The capsules shells used for compounding are exactly the same capsules used in manufacturing and must meet the same strict standards for composition, size, and capacity. Gelatin capsules come in a variety of colors and color combinations as well as dye free (clear). Veggie caps are always clear. A certificate of analysis (C of A) must be supplied with any lot of capsules purchased by a pharmacy. This certificate will document the ingredients used to manufacture the capsule, including any dyes, which may be a concern to patients with allergies to food coloring and additives. The C of A also includes the capsule's expiration date.

Capsules are manufactured in standard sizes that have specific capacities and dimensions. The numbering system for capsule sizes is a bit confusing, because *the smaller the number, the larger the capsule.* Capsules used in human compounding range from size 5 to size 000, with size 5 capsules being very tiny and size 000 being quite large (Figure 6-1).

> **The smaller the number, the larger the capsule.**
> **Size 5: smallest**
> **Size 000: largest**

Capsule shells are composed of a base (body) and a cap. After the capsules are filled, they must be fitted together tightly and "lock." When a bulk container of capsules is opened, the caps and bases will be loosely attached to each other. The compounding procedure includes separating the cap from the base so that the base can be filled with medication. Once filled, the cap will be replaced on the base and locked securely to prevent the capsule from separating before patient administration.

Capsule Filling

The most common way to fill a large quantity of capsules is a precision capsule machine. As discussed in Chapter 3, this machine is size specific or has interchangeable plates and accessories used to fill various sizes of capsules. Precision capsule-filling machines can make 100 or more capsules at a time. The capsules are held upright in the machine, and the body and cap can be separated all at once. The capsules are filled by spreading the prepared powder over the open capsule bases until completely full. The caps are replaced and locked before removing the filled capsule from the machine. There are smaller, manual capsule machines that can make 50 or fewer capsules in one batch (Table 6-1).

There are 2 methods used for settling the powders into the capsule bases when using a capsule machine:

1. The formulated powder is spread across the open capsule bases; the machine is picked up and tapped gently on the counter several times. The remaining powder is spread across the capsule bases again, and the process is repeated until all the powder has been distributed into the open capsules.

2. The other method involves a **tamper** tool. This tool comes in assorted sizes to match the capsule bases. It has plastic or metal pegs that are pushed down into the capsule bases to compress the powders. A small amount of powder is spread over the capsules bases, and the tamper is placed over the open capsules to push the powders down into the bases. This step is repeated until all the powders have been compressed into the capsules (Figure 6-2).

The filling technique required for each formulation should be specified in the master formulation record (MFR) to ensure consistency and correct preparation of the intended formulation. In most cases the powder used will be the API. In some cases a whole tablet or tablets may be placed in a capsule shell and an excipient added. This is known as **overencapsulation**.

If a capsule machine is not available, the traditional hand packing or **"punch" method** can be used. In this method of capsule preparation, the powder(s) prepared from the MFR are piled in a line or rectangle shape where the height of the pile is approximately equal to the depth of the capsule base. Each capsule shell is separated and the technician turns the base upside-down, presses the base into the powder pile to fill it, and then snaps on the cap. This method of capsule filling is time consuming and inaccurate, as it is difficult to get the same amount of powders in each capsule, and each must be filled individually. Because of the difficulty in precise filling, when utilizing the "punch" method, each capsule should be weighed to ensure accuracy (Table 6-2).

Both capsule filling processes can be viewed at various sites on the Internet.

TABLE 6-1 Procedure for Capsule Filling Using a Precision Capsule Machine

Filling Capsules Using a Capsule Machine
Make sure the capsule-making area and machine are clean.
Don appropriate PPE as required.
1. Assemble the capsule machine as directed by the machine manufacturer.
2. Fill the capsule bed by using the orienter (if available) (Figure 6-3). • Make sure capsule bases are in the capsule bed and capsule caps are above the capsule bed. • If no capsule orienter, place each capsules in capsule bed.
3. Separate the capsules per manufacturer instructions. • Set the top tray containing capsule caps off to the side, making sure they stay in the top tray snuggly. • If no capsule separation tray is available, remove capsule caps by hand.
4. Weigh out the ordered API(s) and excipient required for the total amount of capsules necessary to prepare the "batch."
5. Follow the MFR instructions for amounts required in the formulation.
6. Complete the master compounding record. Be sure to have the pharmacist check the weight calculations and the measured amounts of each ingredient required *before mixing*.
7. Use geometric dilution to mix all powders evenly.
8. Make sure capsule bases have "dropped" into capsule bed tray so that capsule bases are even with the tray.
9. Pour a sufficient amount of powder into the capsule bed and spread until all the capsules are filled.
10. Tamp the powder down using either a tamper or the tray lift method.
11. Repeat steps 8 and 9 until *all* the powder has been distributed into the capsule bases.
12. Replace capsule top tray and put the capsules back together per manufacturer instructions. • If no capsule top tray is available, replace capsule tops by hand, making sure they are "locked" together.
13. Remove capsules from capsule top tray per manufacturer instructions or by hand.
14. Dump capsules onto a clean towel and check each capsule to make sure they are locked together.
15. Roll the capsules in the towel to remove any excess powders on the outside of capsules.
16. Finish recording required information on master compounding record.
17. Perform quality assurance procedures listed in MFR. • In most cases this requires weighing a percentage of the finished capsules to make sure they are uniform.
18. Package and label appropriately.
19. Have pharmacist check final product.

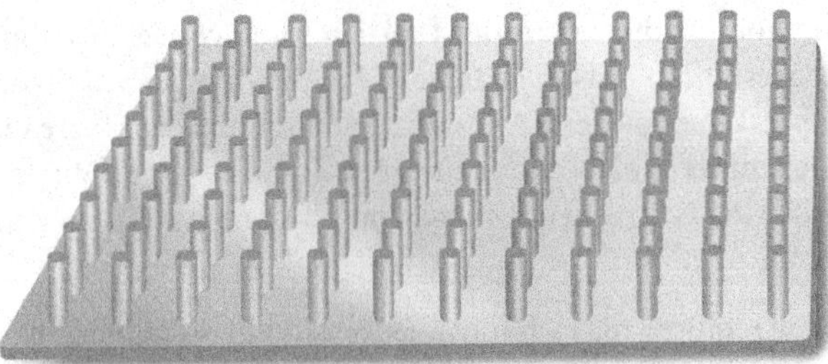

FIGURE 6-2 Capsule tamper.

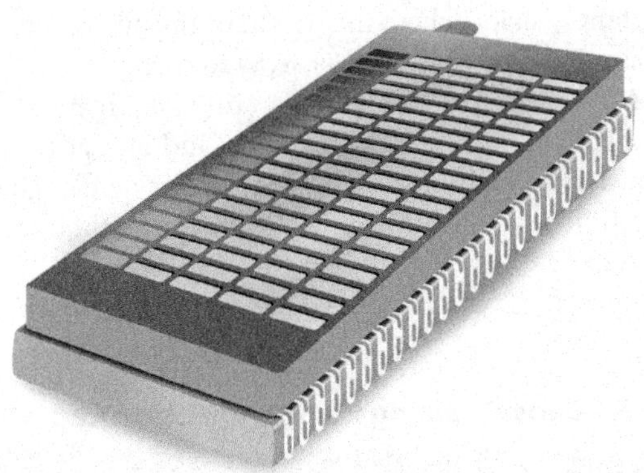

FIGURE 6-3 Capsule orienter.

TABLE 6-2 **Procedure for Filling Capsules Using the "Punch" Method**

Filling Capsules Using the "Punch" Method
1. Make sure capsule making area and supplies are clean.
2. Don appropriate PPE as required.
3. Weigh out all API(s) and excipient ingredients needed to prepare required amount of capsules. Make sure to have enough powder for 1 extra capsule, because there will be some loss during the capsule-filling process.
4. Follow the MFR instructions for amounts needed in the formulation.
5. Complete the master compounding record. Have the pharmacist check the weight calculations and the measured amounts of each ingredient required before mixing.
6. Use geometric dilution to mix all powders evenly.
7. Place the powder mixture for all the capsules on an ointment slab or pad.
8. Using a spatula, arrange the powder into a compact, flat powder bed of uniform thickness.
9. The height of the powder bed should be just slightly shorter than the dimension of the capsule shell base.
10. Separate the capsule caps from the capsule bases.
11. Repeatedly press the open end of the capsule base downward into the bed of powder.
12. Replace the cap on the capsule base loosely and check the weight of the capsule.
13. Add to or remove powder from the capsule shell until the required amount on the MFR is achieved for each capsule.
14. Repeat steps 10-12 until all the powder has been used.
15. Remove any excess powder on the outside of capsules.
16. Finish completing the master compounding record.
17. Package and label appropriately.
18. Have pharmacist check final product.

Excipients (Fillers)

Capsules usually consist of more than 1 ingredient: usually one or more API and an excipient (filler) powder. When a new MFR is written for a compounded capsule, the first step is to find how much of the chosen excipient is required to completely fill the chosen capsule base (100% of the volume). Next, a physical calculation is performed to determine how much of the volume of the capsule base is taken up by the prescribed dose of the active drug(s). Then the *weight of the active drug* is subtracted from the *weight of the excipient* that is needed to fill the capsule. This number is the amount of excipient need in the formulation. The excipient and active powders are then combined and used to evenly fill the capsule bases. Choosing the correct excipient or filler is based on 2 things: compatibility with the active drug and the requirements of the patient. The excipient cannot alter the stability or the profile of the active drug and it should not cause gastric distress or other potential side effects for the patient. Looking at the ingredients in a manufactured dosage form can be a useful tool to identify the excipient that may be used for a compounded formulation. For example, if the drug comes as a manufactured tablet and the package insert lists lactose as an ingredient, lactose can be considered a proper excipient for a compounded capsule. Another excipient, however, should be used for patients with lactose intolerance.

Lactose monohydrate powder is the most common excipient used in compounded capsules. This powder is provided in 2 different types: normal and spray dried (SD). Other common excipients include microcrystalline cellulose, starch, and talc. All of these are USP/NF grades and are generally very stable and nonreactive. Many other materials may be used as fillers to tailor the capsule formulation to the specific patient. There are also some specialized fillers that *must* be used when compounding capsules containing certain drugs. For example, the bioidentical progesterone and testosterone powders used currently in hormone-replacement therapy (HRT) are destroyed by stomach acid. When powder capsules are prepared using these APIs, the drugs are protected by a special excipient called *hypromellose*, which is a specialized form of cellulose developed for this specific purpose. The hypromellose forms a protective ball to surround the active drug protecting it from degradation in the stomach acid.

Mixing Capsule Ingredients

The progesterone and testosterone example discussed in the previous section describes a multi-ingredient capsule. The convenience and ease of administration found in providing a patient's medications all in one "package" is a common reason for prescribing compounded capsules.

Having several ingredients inside 1 capsule makes the *mixing* process a very important step in the preparation. Quality assurance parameters for capsule formulations should always include a check of the powders before they are placed on the capsule machine for spreading into the bases. Most powders are white, so a colored powder is often added to indicate that powders are completely and evenly mixed (homogeneous). This powdered dye is called *powder-dispersion dye or Alum Lake dye.* It is available in a variety of colors. All the powders listed in the MFR are placed in the mixing container and just a "pinch" of the Alum Lake dye is added. The combined powders are mixed until visual inspection shows that the color is evenly distributed throughout the powders. There should not be any visible particles of the dye in the other powders and none of the powder should still be white. The same quality assurance can be attained by assigning a precise amount of time for the mixing process in the procedures section of the MFR.

Powders can be mixed in a special blender, a standard jar, or a simple zip-lock bag. A zip-lock bag is disposable, convenient, and efficient for mixing powders (Table 6-3).

Quality Assurance

Whether you are using a precision capsule machine or a manual method, a quality assurance check is important in all aspects of the capsule preparation process.

All MFRs for capsule formulations must be reviewed and checked by the pharmacist. The amount of each API and excipient, as well as any calculations performed must be checked *before* the formulation is prepared.

TABLE 6-3 Mixing Powders and Dye in a Zip-Lock Bag

1. Place correct amounts of excipient and API powders in a zip-lock bag.
2. Add a "pinch" of Alum Lake dye.
3. Let most of the air out of the bag before sealing.
4. Shake a few times so that you can see the discrete particles of dye as they begin to be dispersed.
5. Shake vigorously to until there are no visible particles of the dye and all the powder is no longer white.
6. Let all the air out of the bag by slightly breaking the seal and lay the bag down on the counter.
7. Manipulate the powders with fingertips to be sure that none of the dye particles remains.

When multiple powders are measured, each powder must be weighed separately. Close the container and place the paper or boat containing the measured powder in front of the container for pharmacist verification. Do this with each powder, even the fillers. Many API containers look alike and drug names on the label may also be similar. This process can ensure that 1 powder was not weighed twice or omitted from the formulation. When all the powders are accurately weighed and have been checked by the pharmacist, add them to the mixing container.

To ensure that the powders and excipients have been distributed evenly through the entire 'batch" of capsules; 10% of the finished capsules (10 of each 100) should be weighed to determine that they are within 5% of the targeted weight. This should be part of the quality assurance checks written into the MFR.

When multiple powders are measured, always weigh each powder separately.

Capsule colors and sizes can be used as a quality assurance tool as well. Some pharmacies may use only one color or size for a specific formulation. For example, a pharmacy may prepare all HRT formulations in red capsules and all pain formulations in blue capsules. This type of color coding can prevent dispensing errors and provide uniformity in the capsule compounding process.

BUD

If there is no stability information available, capsules can be assigned whichever comes *first*:

- The earliest expiration date of any component used in the formulation
- Six months from the date the compound was prepared

TABLETS

Compounded tablets are a unique dosage form not seen in many compounding pharmacy practice because they tend to be quite labor intensive and require special molds and supplies.

There are two basic kinds of compounded tablets:

1. Rapid dissolving tablets (RDTs)
2. Tablet triturates (TTs)

Compounded tablets differ from manufactured tablets in that they are usually not intended to be swallowed. In most cases, compounded tablet dosage forms are placed either on top of or under the tongue, and the drug is absorbed through the mouth's mucous membrane. When preparing solid dosages form, it is important to note that if greater than one-third of the volume of the **cavity** is not base material (active and excipient powders), the dosage form will not bind properly and fall apart. For both of these compressed tablet dosage forms, it is a good idea to write the MFR to make 2 or 3 additional tablets to account for loss during the preparation process.

TABLET TRITURATES

One-Third Displacement Rule

If greater than one-third of the volume of the mold cavity is not base material, the dosage form will not bind properly and fall apart.

Tablet triturates (TTs) are a tiny, durable, sublingual dosage form. They are pressed tablets prepared by compacting the compounded material into an aluminum TT mold that generally has 50 cavities. The cavities are drilled in a flat plate and are calibrated to provide capacities for either 100 or 200 mg. The base of the TT mold has 50 short pegs that correspond to the cavity holes in the plate. The material containing the active drug is pressed into the cavities, and after about 20 minutes, they are pressed out to sit on top of the pegs to dry (Figure 6-4).

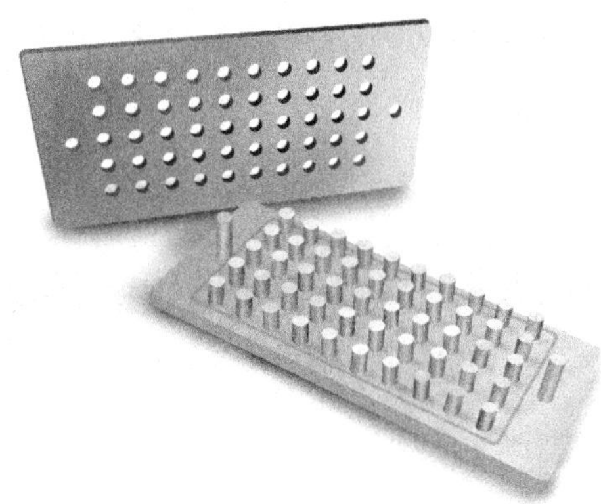

FIGURE 6-4 Triturate mold.

To "punch" the tablet out of the molds:

- Place the cavity tray on the peg platform with the end pegs inserted in the end holes.
- Place index fingers and thumbs on each corner of the cavity tray.
- Apply even, downward pressure on the corners of the cavity tray.
- The cavity tray will drop leaving the tablets behind on the pegs.

Preparation of Tablet Triturates

The base or vehicle used to prepare tablet triturates is a combination of a binder (usually lactose) and a sweetener (sugar). The API is combined with the base mixture in the amounts stated in the MFR. The powders are moistened with a mixture of water and alcohol to form a smooth paste. Tablet triturate material is usually prepared using a mortar and pestle. The proportions of sucrose and lactose in the vehicle mixture can be adjusted to provide a shorter or quicker dissolution of the tablets. The water/alcohol mixture can also be adjusted (Table 6-4).

Video demonstrations of tablet triturate preparation are available on the Internet.

TABLE 6-4 Tablet Triturate Preparation Process

Step 1	Make sure preparation area and supplies are clean.
Step 2	Don appropriate PPE required.
Step 3	Combine API and base in a mortar and pestle.
Step 4	Moisten combined ingredients with a small amount of water and alcohol to form a smooth paste.
Step 5	Press the paste into the specified size mold using a hard plastic spatula.
Step 6	Let the tablets dry for the time period specified in the MFR.
Step 7	Punch damp tablets onto pegs to complete drying. (This may take several hours.)
Step 8	Store in amber pharmacy vial until needed for dispensing.

BUD

If there is no stability information available, tablet triturates can be assigned whichever comes *first*:

- The earliest expiration date of any component used in the formulation
- Six months from the date prepared

RAPID DISSOLVING TABLETS

Rapid dissolving tablets (RDTs) are also pressed tablets but are significantly larger and much more fragile than tablet triturates. These are prepared in a mold made of a block of composite plastic/silicone material that is split to form a top and bottom tray. A typical RDT mold has 36 cavities that can each hold approximately 800 mg of a rapid dissolving tablet formulation. The bottom tray contains the indented cavities and the top block is used as a tamper to compress

TABLE 6-5 Rapid Dissolving Tablets (RDTs) Preparation Process

Step 1	Make sure preparation area and supplies are clean.
Step 2	Don appropriate PPE required.
Step 3	Combine proper amounts of API and base in a mortar and pestle.
Step 4	Compact powders into the bottom tray of cavity molds.
Step 5	Place top tray onto cavity mold to tightly compress powders.
Step 6	Place mold in convection oven and heat for the time and temperature specified in the MFR.
Step 7	Let tablets cool.
Step 8	Package RDTs in individual, airtight blister pack dispensing cards to avoid breakage and water absorption.

the powder tightly into the cavities. Once filled, the mold is placed in a convection oven that provides *dry* heat. This dry heat melts the vehicle to form a tablet that contains the active drug. Once the tablets have been baked, they are removed from the mold and packaged (Table 6-5).

BUD

If there is no stability information available, rapid dissolving tablets can be assigned whichever comes *first*:

- The earliest expiration date of any component used in the formulation
- Six months from the date prepared

TROCHES/LOZENGES

Troches are a popular solid dosage form in compounding pharmacies because they easy to prepare. In addition, if a correction or change to the formulation must be made, the troches can be remelted and an alteration made to the preparation.

Troches deliver medication through mucosal absorption by melting in the cheek pouch (buccal cavity) of the mouth. The saliva created to dissolve the troche should be held in the mouth, not swallowed. Troches are intended to dissolve slowly, usually in 15 to 30 minutes. On rare occasions, a troche will be inserted vaginally.

Troches are made by combining several ingredients. The most common troche vehicle is polyethylene glycol (**PEG**). PEG is a synthetic wax that melts easily, suspends powders well, and cools quickly to become a solid again. PEG itself is very bitter, so the addition of sweetening and flavoring agents is necessary. Most pharmacies use a manufactured, ready-to-melt troche vehicle made from a combination of PEG and a sugar-free sweetener.

The MFR for a troche will reflect the weight of the total amount of the base required to fill the necessary number of cavities, minus the weight of the API(s) and other ingredients such as flavoring. The one-third displacement rule that is used for tablets applies here as well, to ensure the troche firms up correctly.

Reusable molds have nonstick surfaces and separate to release the troches once hardened. Disposable molds allow the troche material to be poured and dispensed in the same container. Most troche molds have 1 g cavities, but 100 mg cavities molds are also available.

The troche vehicle is melted, the medication is added, and the melted material is poured into a mold. When it cools and resolidifies, it can be dispensed like a piece of candy or lozenge. Troches are dispensed in capsule jars or the disposable molds they were prepared in and should be stored in a cool place (Figure 6-5).

BUD

If there is no stability information available, troches can be assigned whichever comes *first*:

- The earliest expiration date of any component used in the formulation
- Six months from the date prepared

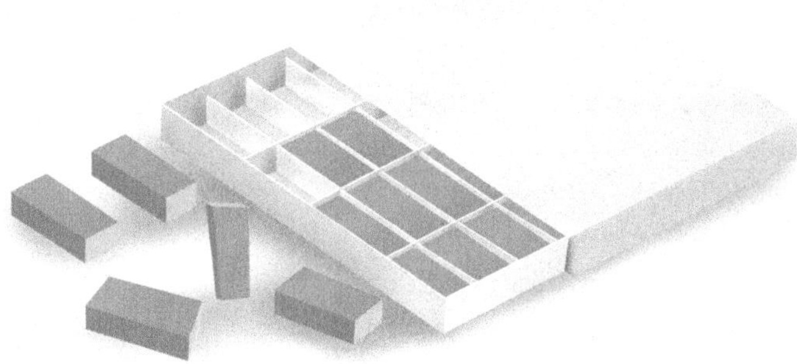

FIGURE 6-5 Disposable troche mold and compounded troches.

LOLLIPOPS

Lollipops are innovative solid dosage forms that are sometimes used to make a medication more appealing, for children. Some pharmacies use candy molds to make lollipops containing medication, but candy molds can vary in capacity, making accuracy a challenge. For a quality medicinal lollipop, the volume of each cavity must be exact in order for the formulation to yield the correct dose of the prescribed drug; therefore a calibrated, precision lollipop mold is the best choice.

Lollipop bases can be a mixture of water and sugar, or corn syrup. Nonreducing sugars are used to create sugar-free lollipops. The syrupy mixture is heated to a high temperature using a hot plate or stirring hot plate. A thermometer is needed so that the mixture reaches the precise temperature (known as the "hard-crack" stage), so that when it cools, it is becomes a solid. Once the water has evaporated, the active drug and flavoring are added to the syrup and poured into the mold.

Preparing lollipops from syrup is time consuming and labor intensive because of the "cooking" process required to reach the required temperature. Many pharmacies will opt to make "troches on stick" that are much easier to prepare and in most cases provide an equivalent delivery of drug.

BUD

If there is no stability information available, lollipops can be assigned whichever comes *first*:

- The earliest expiration date of any component used in the formulation
- Six months from the date prepared

Suppositories

Suppositories are solid, molded dosage forms that may be inserted in the rectum, vagina, or urethra. The medication delivered in suppositories is absorbed through the mucous membranes of these body cavities.

Suppository Vehicles

There are two primary types of vehicles used to compound suppositories:

1. Plant oils: melts at body temperature
2. PEG: dissolves in body fluid

PEG-based vehicles must have water to dissolve. In addition PEG-based suppositories are naturally going to pull moisture from the mucous membrane to dissolve, causing irritation in many patients. PEG vehicles are a standard mixture of PEG 400 (a liquid) and PEG 8000 (a very hard solid). Pharmacies can either purchase these 2 forms of PEG and make their own combination, or purchase a manufactured, ready-to-use blend.

TABLE 6-6 Suppository Preparation Process

Step 1	Make sure preparation area and supplies are clean.
Step 2	Don appropriate PPE required.
Step 3	Melt the suppository vehicle to a liquid.
Step 4	Sprinkle the API powders required for the formulation by the MFR into the melted vehicle.
Step 5	Stir thoroughly.
Step 6	Pour the combined vehicle and API into the mold.
Step 7	Cool at room temperature until the mixture hardens.
Step 8	Store finished formulations in the refrigerator (if needed).

Cocoa butter is the traditional plant oil used in melting suppository formulations; however, cocoa butter scorches easily and does not resolidify if overheated. Fatty blends, made from palm kernel oil, are easier to work with and will come in either a solid mass or as small formed pellets called *pastilles*.

The amounts listed in the MFR are based on the weight of the volume of the suppository vehicle (the density factor). Like the other dosage forms in this chapter, the one-third displacement rule must be applied so that when the melted materials return to a solid form, the suppository will not break apart when administered. The method of preparation is the same regardless of which suppository base is used (Table 6-6).

Suppository Molds

Reusable suppository molds have a 2 g capacity. They are made of aluminum or plastic and can make from 10 to 100 suppositories at a time. Like a reusable troche mold, the cavity strips of a reusable suppository mold are bound together with springs and bolts that are loosened to allow for easy release from the mold (Figure 6-6).

Disposable suppository molds come in a variety of sizes and are made of a light gauge plastic or rubber. They have a fill line or ridge that marks the correct capacity level for the size being prepared. The suppositories can be formed and dispensed in the same container and are packaged as a strip of connected cavities (Figure 6-7).

The standard, bullet-shaped molds are used for both rectal and vaginal suppositories. A urethral suppository mold has a more tubular shape to ease insertion into the urethra.

Suppository Preparation

In both a disposable or reusable mold the suppository material should be overpoured, because as the suppository material cools, it will contract into the mold. Any excess that is left after cooling can be trimmed away with a spatula or razor knife.

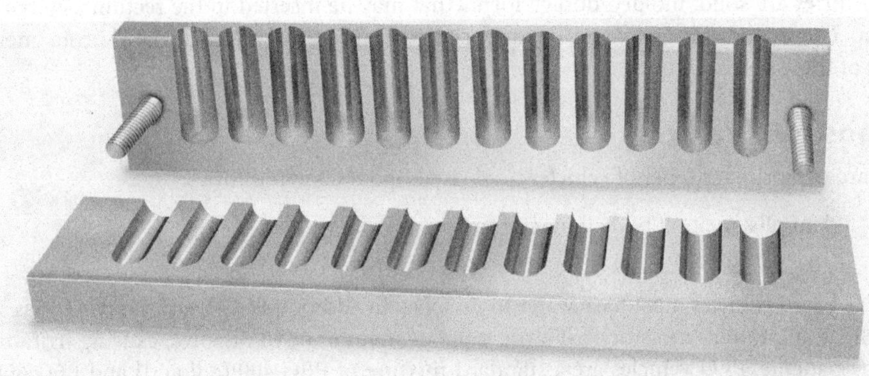

FIGURE 6-6 Reusable suppository molds.

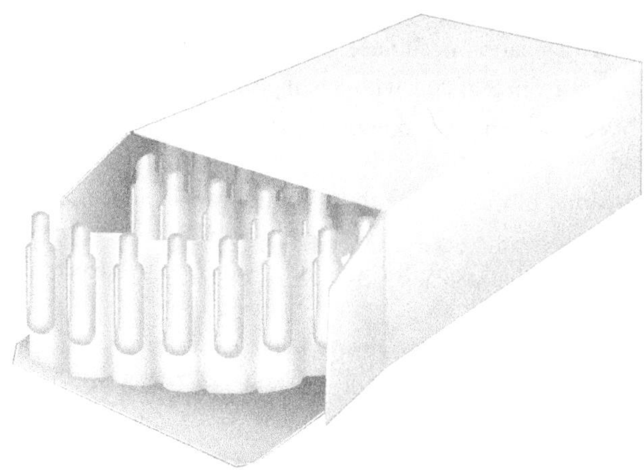

FIGURE 6-7 Disposable suppository molds.

BUD

If there is no stability information available, suppositories can be assigned whichever comes *first*:

- The earliest expiration date of any component used in the formulation
- Six months from the date prepared

Lip Balms

Compounded lip balms are often prescribed to deliver antiviral medications and sunscreen. This unique dosage form can be formulated for use on more than just lips. Dermaceuticals can also be prepared for topical application to blemishes or other areas. Lip balm bases are a mixture of PEG molecular weights or melting vehicles derived from plant oils. Ready-to-use lip balm bases are also available. Plant oil bases are the preferable base because they are not bitter tasting or absorb moisture like a PEG vehicle. Flavoring agents can be added to either type to increase palatability and patient compliance. Lip balms are usually dispensed in a 5 g tube applicator. These tubes have a twist up piston on the bottom and a cap on the top.

BUD

If there is no stability information available, lip balms can be assigned whichever comes *first*:

- The earliest expiration date of any component used in the formulation
- Six months from the date prepared

CONCLUSION

Preparing solid dosage forms is a unique and innovative way to combine APIs into a complete package that may not otherwise be available. A technician proficient in solid dosage form compounding preparation will enhance the ability of a pharmacy to provide patients with a convenient, quality-compounded dosage form designed to increase patient compliance and satisfaction.

CHAPTER SUMMARY

- Solid dosage forms offer sustained stability and the ability to combine several drugs into one product.
- Capsules are used to deliver medication to the stomach for absorption through the GI tract or as a container for the correct dose of a medication.

- Capsules are made of gelatin or cellulose.
- Capsules sizes range from 5 to 000, with 5 being the smallest and 000 the largest size.
- Capsules are filled with either a precision capsule machine or by hand using the "punch" method.
- Lactose monohydrate powder is the most common excipient used in compounded capsules.
- Ten percent of the finished capsules should be weighed to determine that they are within 5% of the targeted weight.
- When measuring multiple powders, always weigh each powder separately.
- Tablet triturates (TTs) and rapid dissolving tablets (RDTs) are compounded solid dosage forms.
- Compounded tablet dosage forms are placed either on top of or under the tongue and the drug is absorbed through the mouth's mucous membrane.
- Both TTs and RDTs are absorbed through the mouth's mucous membrane.
- Troches deliver medication through mucosal absorption by melting in the cheek pouch (buccal cavity) of the mouth.
- Lollipops are innovative solid dosage forms that are sometimes used to make a medication more appealing.
- Preparing lollipops is time consuming and labor intensive because of the "cooking" process required to reach the required temperature.
- Suppositories are solid, molded dosage forms that may be inserted in the rectum, vagina, or urethra.
- Suppository vehicles are composed of either plant oils or PEG.
- The "one-third displacement rule" applies to most solid dosage forms.
- Compounded lip balms are often prescribed to deliver antiviral medications and sunscreen.
- Dermaceuticals can also be prepared for topical application to blemishes or other areas.

PTCB Review Questions

1. Which of the following statements are *false*?
   A. Compounded lip balms are prescribed to deliver antiviral medications.
   B. Lip balms can only be formulated for use on lips.
   C. Lollipop bases can be a mixture of water and corn syrup.
   D. Flavoring and sweetening agents should be added to troches.
2. What vehicle is commonly used in compounding suppositories?
   A. Water
   B. Lactose
   C. PEG or plant oils
   D. Corn syrup
3. Which of the following statements are *true*?
   A. Beyond-use dating is not important for solid dosage form.
   B. PEG is never used in compounding troches.
   C. The medication delivered in suppositories is absorbed through the mucous membranes of these body cavities.
   D. RDTs must be prepared using a microwave oven.
4. What is the most common excipient used in capsule preparation?
   A. Lactose monohydrate powder
   B. PEG 1450
   C. Plant oil
   D. Hypromellose

5. Which solid dosage forms are absorbed through the mucous membrane?
   A. Vaginal suppositories
   B. Tablet triturates
   C. Lollipops
   D. Both A and B
6. Which of the following statements are *true*?
   A. The "punch" method is the most precise way to fill capsules.
   B. Suppositories are prepared the same way using either base vehicle.
   C. PEG bases used in suppositories do not need any water to dissolve.
   D. Lollipop bases must be heated at low temperature.
7. Why would a capsule be the best choice for a patient?
   A. The correct dose is not available in a manufactured product.
   B. To omit an excipient this is found in manufactured versions of the drug.
   C. For delivery of multiple drugs in one capsule.
   D. All of the above.
8. Which solid dosage form requires dry heat in its preparation?
   A. RDTs
   B. Lip balm
   C. TTs
   D. Troches
9. Which vehicle used in compounding solid dosage forms melts at body temperature?
   A. Lactose
   B. PEG
   C. Plant oils
   D. TTs
10. The "one-third displacement rule" applies to which compounded solid dosage forms?
    A. RDT
    B. TT
    C. Troches and suppositories
    D. All of the above

Techs in Practice: Discussion Topics and Questions

SCENARIO 1

Your class or compounding facility is in need of a new capsule machine. Research different manufactures products and present the pros and cons of each manufacture's product to your coworkers or classmates. Make a recommendations for 2 products that will best suite your facility's needs, and why.

SCENARIO 2

The pharmacy you are employed at is interested in starting to prepare solid dosage forms.

Based on this chapter, which two formulations would you recommend they start preparing? Give several reasons for each of your choices.

Lab 1

Design a quality-control process using color coding for the different types of capsules a pharmacy may prepare.

Lab 2

Prepare 5 capsules using the procedures in Table 6-2.

Follow quality assurance measures for accuracy.

Time the process and come up with two ways to improve accuracy and decrease preparation time.

Calculation Review Questions

A prescription is for diazepam 10 mg suppositories. You need to compound 30 suppositories. The density factor of a melting suppository base is 1.82 for a 2 g mold. This means that a 2 g mold holds 1.82 g of the suppository base. Suppose you are using 2 g suppository molds to prepare the medication in the prescription.

1. What amount of the suppository vehicle must be measured to fill thirty 2 g molds?

A batch of 100 capsules has been prepared. The final quality check is to verify that all the capsules weigh within 5% (±) of the target weight of 54.2 mg. 10 capsules have been chosen at random and they have the following weights: 55.1 mg, 54.99 mg, 56.01 mg, 54.5 mg, 51.2 mg, 54.6 mg, 55.2 mg, 57.9 mg, 56.7 mg, and 55.4 mg.

2. What is the range of acceptable weights for this target weight?
3. Are any of the capsules listed outside of that 5% range?
4. If so, which ones?

This chapter includes the following PTCE Blueprint Knowledge Areas

Section 1.0-1.4 Strengths/dose, dosage forms, physical appearance, routes of administration, and duration of drug therapy.

Section 2.0-2.6 Record keeping, documentation, and retention (eg, length of time prescriptions are maintained on file).

Section 2.0-2.11 Infection control standards (eg, laminar air flow, clean room, hand washing, cleaning counting trays, countertop, and equipment). (OSHA, USP/NF Chapter ⟨795⟩ and ⟨797⟩)

Section 2.0-2.13 Professional standards regarding the roles and responsibilities of pharmacist, pharmacy technicians, and other pharmacy employees. (TJC, BOP)

Section 2.0-2.15 Facility, equipment, and supply requirements (eg, space requirements, prescription file storage, cleanliness, reference materials). (TJC, USP, BOP)

Section 3.0-3.3 Documentation (eg, batch preparation, compounding record).

Section 3.0-3.5 Selection and use of equipment and supplies.

Section 3.0-3.7 Non-sterile compounding processes.

Section 6.0-6.3 Calculate dosing required.

Section 6.0-6.4 Fill process (eg, select appropriate product, apply special handling requirements, measure and prepare product for final check).

Section 6.0-6.5 Labeling requirements (eg, auxiliary and warning labels, expiration date, patient specific information).

Section 6.0-6.7 Dispensing process (eg, validation, documentation, and distribution).

Section 7.0-7.4 Storage requirements (eg, refrigeration, freezer, warmer).

This chapter includes the following Ex-CPT Test Specifications

Section 1 A-4 Comply with rules and regulations when filling prescriptions.

Section 1 A-6 Maintain a clean work environment in the pharmacy and patient care areas.

Section 1 C-7 Properly package prescription medication in child-resistant containers or other approved containers as required.

Section 1 C-8 Comply with professional, state, and federal laws and regulations.

Section 1 C-9 Use information found on medication stock bottles, such as drug name and strength, expiration date, and lot number.

Section 2 A-2 Differentiate among various dosage forms (eg, tablets vs capsules, ointment vs creams, controlled release vs immediate release, parenteral vs oral).

Section 2 B-1 Interpret basic medical terminology commonly used in the pharmacy in order to effectively assist the pharmacist.

Section 3 B-2 Identify drugs that require special handling procedures.

Section 3 B-5 Follow proper record keeping procedures pertaining to the pharmacy.

Section 3 B-6 Follow the pharmacy's quality assurance policies and procedures.

Section 3 B-14 Properly and accurately prepare prescription labels.

Section 3 B-18 Use auxiliary labels properly.

Section 3 B-19 Properly label drug products packaged in approved containers or, when appropriate, original packages.

Section 3 C-2 Calculate the quantities of prescription medications to be dispensed.
Section 3 C-4 Properly calculate individual and daily dosages.
Section 3 D-1 Follow proper compounding procedures for non-sterile products.
Section 3 D-3 Properly repackage and label unit of use products.
Section 3 D-4 Properly calculates expiration dates for repackaged products.

This chapter includes the following ASHP Model Curriculum for Pharmacy Technician Training Goal Statements, Objectives, and Instructional Objectives

OBJ 2.4 Efficiently secures information to complete a prescription/medication order.
OBJ 3.3 Follow established laws and protocols to select the appropriate product.
OBJ 3.5 Accurately count or measure finished dosage forms as specified by the prescription/medication order.
OBJ 3.6 Collect the correct ingredients for sterile or non-sterile products that require compounding.
OBJ 3.7 Accurately determine the correct amounts of ingredients for a compounded product.
OBJ 3.11 Follow safety policies and procedures in the preparation of all medications.
OBJ 3.13 Package the product in the appropriate type and size of container using a manual process or automated system.
OBJ 3.14 Follow an established manual procedure or electronic procedure to generate accurate and complete product labels.
OBJ 3.18 Follow established policies and procedures for recording the preparation of bulk, unit dose, and special doses of medications prepared for immediate or in anticipation of future use.
OBJ 3.19 Follow the manufacturer's recommendation and/or the pharmacy's guidelines for storage of all medications prior to distribution.
OBJ 12.1 Follow policies and procedures for sanitation management, hazardous waste handling, and infection control.
OBJ 12.3 Maintain a clean and neat work environment.
OBJ 35.1 Apply the principles of quality assurance to all technician activities.

Answers to PTCB Questions

1. **B**
2. **C**
3. **C**
4. **A**
5. **D**
6. **B**
7. **D**
8. **A**
9. **C**
10. **D**

Answers to Calculation Questions

1. 54.6 g
2. 51.5 to 56.9 mg
3. Yes
4. 57.9 mg and 51.2 mg

CHAPTER 7

Semisolid Dosage Forms

INTRODUCTION

In modern compounding, placing medications into specialized, semisolid vehicles is an area of great innovation in serving individual patient needs. The practice of delivering medications to the muscles, tissue, or the bloodstream provides doctors and pharmacists with a variety of treatment options.

KEY TERMS

Analgesic: A medication that relieves pain

Cream: A semisolid, stable emulsion of water and oil that is applied to the skin

Emulsion: A stable, homogeneous mixture of oil and water

Gel: Thickened liquid

Hydrophilic: Readily absorbing or dissolving in water, water loving

Luer lock (LL): A standardized system of small-scale fluid fittings, which prevents leaks between connections of hypodermic syringe tips and needles

Liposome: A microscopic artificial sac composed of fatty substances that can be used as a vehicle for administration of nutrients and medications

Lotion: A semisolid, stable emulsion of water and oil that is applied to the skin and has less viscosity (less thin) than a cream

Occlusive: Preventing the penetration of water or air

Ointment: A semisolid material that is applied externally to the skin or to mucous membrane

Phospholipid: A lipid component of cell membranes

Stable: To stay mixed or together, unchanging or fixed

Systemic absorption: An effect that takes place at a location beyond the initial point of contact, affecting the entire body and not just locally

Topical: Applied to the surface of skin to treat a local condition of the skin surface

Transdermal (TD): Across or through the skin

LEARNING OBJECTIVES

- Describe the types of semisolid dosage forms.
- Explain the steps in preparing a semlsolid dosage form.
- Explain the differences between transdermal and topical delivery formulations.
- Describe the vehicles used for compounding semisolid formulations.
- List the common solvents used in semisolid compounded medications.
- Explain how transdermal medications are delivered.
- List the sources of drug used in topical and transdermal formulations.
- Describe the methods and devices used to compound and dispense semisolid formulations.
- Explain the importance of quality assurance measures for semisolid dosage forms.
- Explain the parameters for beyond-use dating for each semisolid dosage forms.

TABLE 7-1 Steps to Preparing Semisolid Compounds

1. Identify an appropriate published formulation or write a new master formulation record (MFR) for the preparation.
2. Don appropriate PPE and clean the preparation area and equipment.
3. Accurately weigh and/or measure the ingredients.
4. Have all ingredients collected, amounts to be used determined, and calculations completed before beginning the preparation.
5. Thoroughly mix the active ingredient(s) with a suitable solvent.
6. Choose the proper vehicle.
7. Prepare the medication.
8. Document the process and specific ingredients on the master compounding record (MCR).
9. Follow appropriate quality assurance parameters in the MCR and MFR.
10. Have the pharmacist check the final product.

FORMULATIONS

The most common semisolid formulations include the following:

- Creams
- Lotions
- Gels
- Ointments

Active medication ingredients are delivered via a semisolid formulation in one of two ways:

> ***Topical*** **medications are used to treat the skin.**
> ***Transdermal (TD)*** **medications are used to deliver the drug past the skin into the bloodstream, muscle, or tissue.**

1. **Topical** route: Applied to the surface of the skin to treat a local condition
2. **Transdermal (TD)** route: Penetrates past the skin to treat tissue or to enter the bloodstream for a systemic effect

All semisolid formulations are prepared using the basic steps listed in Table 7-1. It is important to remember that *all* calculations, active pharmaceutical ingredients (APIs), solvents, and vehicles *must be checked by the pharmacist before* any compounding begins.

SOLVENTS

Active drugs and other powders incorporated into compounded medications to be applied topically, should be in *solution*, or be able to dissolve in the vehicle. This makes the drug more absorbable into normal skin. A solution is formed when a solvent is added to a solute and the liquid and powder become one homogeneous mixture.

Different APIs require different solvents. This is an important consideration in any compounded formulation, because the vehicle, the solvent, and the drug all have to work together to achieve an accurate final product. Many formulations require a combination of active drugs and each drug requires a suitable solvent. In other words, a formulation with multiple drugs will have multiple solvents. The correct solvent will be included in the master formulation record (MFR) written for the formulation. Sometimes a powder is *suspended* in an **ointment** being used to treat the skin, but the powders going into a **cream** should always be in solution before going into the vehicle (Table 7-2).

> ***All*** **ingredients and calculations** ***must*** **be checked by the pharmacist** ***before*** **any compounding begins.**

VEHICLES

The correct vehicle is chosen based on how the drug is to be delivered (either topically or transdermally) and its intended purpose. The compounding pharmacist will use their knowledge and judgment to evaluate the drug(s) and indication(s) in order to choose which vehicle is most appropriate to deliver the prescribed medication.

In most cases, it is not appropriate to use a transdermal vehicle for a topical application. For example, lidocaine, applied to the face in order to numb the skin, should not be transported across the skin into the bloodstream. On the other hand, if the cream is being used to deliver

TABLE 7-2 Common Solvents Use in Semisolid Formulations

Common Solvents
Water
Alcohol
Oil

hormones into the bloodstream for **systemic absorption**, it is imperative to choose a transdermal vehicle because a topical vehicle may not perform properly.

Creams

Topical creams are prescribed to treat local skin conditions, a disruption of normal skin, or to anesthetize the skin. *Transdermal* creams are prescribed to deliver **analgesics** and other medications into the bloodstream or tissues and muscles.

Creams are a semisolid, opaque mixture of oil and water and in most cases are applied to the skin. If you have ever made salad dressing, you know that oil and water can be mixed by vigorous shaking, but a few minutes after you put the bottle down, the 2 components separate. A cream has additional ingredients added to the oil and water mixture to cause the 2 parts to stay together for a long time, the same way that a store-bought, creamy dressing remains a **stable** mixture until the expiration date. This stabilized mixture of oil and water, or one that does not separate, is called an **emulsion**.

Creams can be *water-in-oil* emulsions, which means they contain more oil than water and remain *on* the skin. Cold cream, designed to smooth skin and remove makeup, is an example of this type of emulsion. *Oil-in-water* emulsions (contain more water than oil) are more common. Instead of remaining on the skin, these emulsions are *absorbed into* the skin. There is a noticeable difference when each type is applied to the skin. The water-in-oil cream mixture leaves the skin feeling greasy and takes longer to be absorbed, whereas the oil-in-water emulsion is absorbed very quickly, leaving the skin feeling moist. Most drugs and common solvents can be incorporated into either type of emulsion.

Being familiar with the variety of options available in cream vehicles can be very beneficial to providing the best product to a patient. For example, a specific vehicle may be chosen for a patient that has sensitivity to certain ingredients. Some vehicles may be chosen based on where the medication needs to be applied, like under the arms or the genitals. Manufactured compounding cream vehicles are carefully designed to enhance the efficiency of the compounding process. These manufactured cream vehicles have tested stability giving them an extremely long shelf life when they are stored appropriately.

BUD and Storage

If there is no stability information available, creams can be assigned whichever comes *first*:

- The earliest expiration date of any component used in the formulation
- Thirty days from the date prepared

If an antibiotic is included in the formulation, the suggested BUD is whichever comes first:

- Fourteen days
- Course of therapy

Lotions

A **lotion** is a pourable water-in-oil emulsion intended for application to the skin. Lotions are thin versions of cream. In general, they do not deliver medication transdermally; however, a transdermal cream is sometimes thinned to the consistency of a lotion, and it can still retain transdermal properties. Lotions are often used when a medication needs to be applied over a large area of the skin because a thinner emulsion is easier to spread over the body surface. Also, if drugs contained in the medication are in suspension, a lotion can be easily remixed. Lotions also provide moisturizing properties and vanish into the skin.

BUD and Storage

If there is no stability information available, lotions can be assigned whichever comes *first*:

- The earliest expiration date of any component used in the formulation
- Thirty days from the date prepared

Keep away from heat.

Ointments and Gels

Some topical vehicles are **occlusive**, which means they provide a barrier from water and air. The most common occlusive is an ointment, which is a semisolid mixture that does not contain water. Because of the high oil content, ointments also have moisturizing properties. Occlusive ointments and **gels** are used to deliver the medication to a specific local area of skin. At the same time, ointments provide protection by holding in the natural moisture of the skin. The best-known occlusive ointment is *petrolatum*, commonly called Vaseline. *Petrolatum, White NF* is commonly used in compounding. Drugs having oil solubility can be incorporated into petrolatum and drugs not soluble in oil are suspended in the ointment.

Other occlusive vehicles include **hydrophilic** petrolatum and hydrophilic ointment (PEG ointment). Both of these vehicles are ointments, so they are oil miscible. Hydrophilic petrolatum is also miscible with water. Hydrophilic ointment is miscible with both water and alcohol (Table 7-3).

Some gel vehicles also have occlusive properties (Table 7-4). For example, poloxamer gel remains on the skin and provides some protection from air and water. Poloxamer gels were created as the vehicle for PLO (Pluronic lecithin organo) gel, the original transdermal compounding vehicle.

BUD and Storage (Ointment)

If there is no stability information available, ointments can be assigned whichever comes *first*:

- The earliest expiration date of any component used in the formulation
- Six months from the date prepared

Keep away from heat.

TABLE 7-3 Ointment Vehicle Properties

Ointments Vehicles	Properties
Petrolatum	Oil miscible Occlusive
Hydrophilic ointment	Oil miscible Water miscible Alcohol miscible Occlusive
Hydrophilic petrolatum	Oil miscible Water miscible Occlusive

TABLE 7-4 Gel Vehicle Properties

Gel Vehicles	Properties
Poloxamer gel	Occlusive Get thicker as it warms Used for transdermal PLO gel Water miscible Alcohol miscible
Anhydrous gel	Contains no water
Carbomer gel	Contains water (or alcohol and water) Thins as it warms

BUD and Storage (Gel)

If there is no stability information available, gels can be assigned whichever comes *first*:

- The earliest expiration date of any component used in the formulation
- Anhydrous gel: 6 months from the date prepared
- Carbomer or poloxamer gel: 30 days from the date prepared

Keep away from heat.

It is important to choose a vehicle that will work with all the ingredients required for the formulation. For example, a combination of salicylic acid and urea is often prescribed to treat warts. Salicylic acid is soluble in alcohol whereas urea is soluble in water. Using Table 7-4, we can see that hydrophilic ointment is miscible with both solvents, making it the best vehicle for this preparation.

TRANSDERMALS

Transdermal (TD) medications are delivered via liposomes on the skin. A **liposome** is a microscopic, fluid-filled pouch whose walls are made of layers of **phospholipids** identical in makeup to the phospholipids that make up cell membranes. Liposomes are an extremely efficient way to deliver substances to the bloodstream and cells. The liposomes in the transdermal vehicle "unite" with the liposomes in the skin creating a group of similar cells that then carry the drug through the skin into the capillary bed or tissue and muscle beneath the skin. A transdermal vehicle is used to deliver the drug into the bloodstream or to nerves and receptors in the tissue beyond the skin.

Transdermal vehicles are generally oil-in-water emulsions chosen for their ability to "push" the drug past the skin into the capillary bed or tissue and muscle. The first transdermal vehicle developed to provide transdermal absorption was PLO gel. PLO gel is an oil-in-water emulsion of plant phospholipids and poloxamer gel. It was developed in the late 1990s by pharmacists looking for innovative ways to deliver medications through the skin. It leaves the poloxamer gel behind and carries the drug across the skin using liposomes that are absorbed into the skin.

Although PLO gel represented an incredibly innovative drug delivery system, new and improved versions of vehicles that provide liposomal penetration enhancement are now used more frequently. Newer transdermal vehicles have increased stability, moisturizing properties, and are thicker than the PLO gel. This allows for more active ingredients to be incorporated into the formulation. The use of transdermal vehicles is accepted in a growing number of medical and pharmacy practices. It has been especially successful in hormone therapy. Hormones can be dissolved and placed in liposomal vehicles and delivered to thin skinned areas of the body such as the wrist, underarms, inner thighs, or back of the knee, increasing levels in the blood. Blood levels are continuously monitored and the dose can be titrated to the target hormone level for the patient. Transdermal creams are also now often used to deliver complex combinations of pain medications.

SOURCE OF DRUG

As in the preparation of other dosage forms discussed, there are 2 main sources for the drugs that are included in topical and transdermal medications.

1. Prepared dosage forms (tablets, capsules, and injection solutions)
2. API powders

The simplest compounded topical medications are prepared by combining 2 commercially available creams, ointments, gels, or lotions. The technician needs to use dilution techniques and calculate the concentrations of each separate ingredient in order to prepare these formulations.

METHODS OF PREPARATION

Many of the compounding techniques we have discussed in previous chapters are also used in the preparation of compounded creams, ointments, gels, and lotions. When preparing a semisolid compound manually, the technician uses the particle reduction, levigation, and geometric dilution techniques discussed in Chapter 4. Instead of a beaker or graduate and

TABLE 7-5 Process for Manually Preparing a Semisolid Compound from Prepared Ointments

1. Don appropriate PPE and clean the preparation area and equipment.
2. Weigh out both ointments in appropriate volumes for the mixture as indicated on the MFR.
3. Fill out the MCR and have the pharmacist check all calculations, ingredients, and volumes before mixing.
4. Using an ointment slab and a spatula, combine the 2 ointments together using geometric dilution by continuously pressing one ointment into the other until both products are well integrated.
5. Do quality assurances checks as instructed in the MFR.
6. Transfer final product into an appropriate size ointment jar.
7. Label appropriately as instructed in the MFR.
8. Get a final check by the pharmacist and complete the MCR.

TABLE 7-6 Process for Manually Preparing Semisolid Formulations with Multiple Active Ingredients and "QS AD"

1. Don appropriate PPE and clean the preparation area and equipment.
2. Weigh each active powder detailed in the MFR (if using prepared dosage forms, count out appropriate number of tablets or capsules).
3. Fill out MCR and have the pharmacist check to ensure all calculations, ingredients, and amounts are correct.
4. Reduce and triturate the active powders in an appropriate mortar and pestle.
5. Add the required solvent to the active powders and mix to form a smooth paste or solution as instructed in the MFR.
6. Using a rubber spatula, remove the powder and solvent mixture from the mortar and pestle and place in a clean, tared weigh boat or weigh paper on the balance.
7. Add the cream vehicle to the mixture on the balance, until the balance displays the proper final volume.
8. Remove entire mixture (active powder/solvent mixture, and cream vehicle) from the balance.
9. Place back into the mortar or onto an ointment slab or ointment paper.
10. Continue mixing ingredients until a homogeneous mixture is achieved.
11. Do quality assurance checks as instructed by the MFR.
12. Transfer final formulation to an appropriate ointment jar or dispensing device.
13. Label appropriately as directed by the MFR.
14. Finish filling out the MCR and get a final pharmacist check.

a stir rod used for a liquid preparation, a spatula and an ointment slab, or a large mortar and pestle set is used. These formulations can be as simple as mixing 2 ointments or creams together, or much more complex when active drug(s) are included as powders into the preparation (Table 7-5).

Frequently, the MFR will use the term "QS AD" to indicate the amount of vehicle to be used in the preparation. Table 7-6 describes the process of preparing a formulation using multiple active ingredients and QS AD.

MIXING DEVICES

Many electronic devices have been developed to help make the semisolid compounding process more efficient. These devices eliminate much of the labor involved in mixing ingredients and packaging medication formulations for dispensing.

Electronic Mortar and Pestle

An electronic mortar and pestle (EMP) (see Chapter 3) is used for preparing semisolid dosage forms. The machine has a small, powerful motor that turns a shaft and mixing blade, like a drill turns a drill bit. An EMP uses specialized jars manufactured in standard sizes. Each jar has a bottom that fits tightly enough to prevent leaking but that pushes up inside the jar to move creams toward the top. The jar lids have a threaded nipple in their center that is used to connect the jar to the machine by screwing it into a movable arm. The jar is attached to the arm, and the time and speed are chosen from the display screen. When the machine starts its process, the blade spins inside the jar and the arm moves up and down. When the EMP is used, particle reduction, levigation, and geometric dilution steps can be skipped because the machine performs these actions. In addition, the EMP jar that the product was mixed in can be dispensed to the patient, or special attachments can be used to transfer the finished formulation into another dispensing container or device (Figure 7-1). The process for preparing a semisolid formulation using an EMP is listed in Table 7-7.

Tips for preparing formulations using an EMP

- Always place some of the vehicle in the jar ***first***. This will keep the powders from sticking to the sides or bottom of the jar and ensure they are mixed evenly throughout the preparation.
- Although the jars are opaque, a visual check should be done to be sure the formulation is the proper color and that there is no separation of the cream.
- A small amount of the preparation should be rubbed between the finger and thumb to make sure there is no grittiness that would indicate undissolved powder particles.

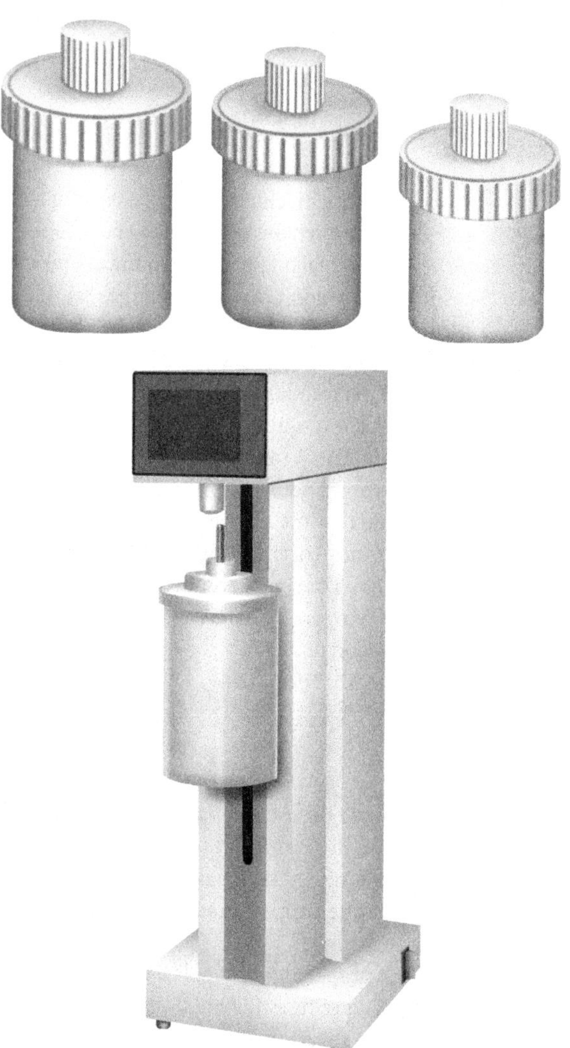

FIGURE 7-1 EMP jars and EMP. (*Reproduced with permission from Unguator Technology.*)

TABLE 7-7 Process for Preparing a Semisolid Formulation Using an EMP

1. Don appropriate PPE and clean the preparation area and equipment properly.
2. Weigh the powders individually as instructed in the MFR.
3. Fill out the MCR and have the pharmacist check all calculations, ingredients, and volumes before mixing.
4. Place the EMP jar on the balance.
5. Tare the balance after placing the jar on the pan.
6. Place a portion of the cream vehicle in the jar.
7. Place alcohol soluble drugs in the jar.
8. Place the solvent being used for these powders in the jar.
9. Place additional cream vehicle in the jar.
10. Place the water-soluble drugs in the jar.
11. Add the required water to wet the water-soluble powders to the EMP jar.
12. Keep adding cream vehicle until the balance displays the total volume to be prepared.
13. Remove jar with mixture from the balance.
14. Place the proper lid on the EMP jar.
15. Connect the jar to the EMP per manufactures instructions.
16. Choose correct time and speed to complete proper mixing per the MFR.
17. Do all quality assurance checks included in the MFR.
18. Label the EMP jar appropriately as directed by the MFR.
19. Finish filling out the MCR and get a final check by the pharmacist.

Ointment Mills

An ointment mill (Fig. 3-25) is another machine that is used to mix creams, ointments, gels, and lotions in compounding pharmacies. The mill mechanism consists of a set of three ceramic rollers powered by a powerful motor and gears. The center roller is stationary. The back and front rollers can be adjusted independently to be closer or farther away from the center roller. All 3 rollers turn together, at the same speed. The machine is equipped with a large red safety button that can be used to stop the machine if something gets stuck inside the rollers. There is a "free-wheel" knob that is used to turn the rollers manually for proper cleaning and maintenance. Semisolid preparations are laid out on the back roller and the rotation of the rollers pushes the material around the middle roller and over the front roller and out onto an attached tray. Preparations are sometimes done in a 2-step process using both the ointment mill and the EMP. First, the preparation is mixed by the EMP in an EMP jar. Then the cream is squirted on to the back roller of the ointment mill and processed through the rollers for final mixing. Instructional demonstration videos of the mixing processes for both the EMP and an ointment mill are available on the Internet.

Using proper technique, an experienced pharmacy technician can provide quality and precisely dosed medication in compounded creams, ointments, gels, and lotions, using an electric mixing device or with just a spatula and a mortar and pestle.

PRECISION DISPENSING CONTAINERS AND DEVICES

Traditionally, creams and ointments have been dispensed either in jars with tight fitting lids or in tubes. It is difficult to get a precise dose amount out of a tube or jar because the patient does not have an accurate way of measuring. In most cases, the patient will immerse a finger in the jar to remove product, or squeeze some from a tube. Today, a variety of precise dispensing devices are available to ensure proper dosing.

The syringe-to-syringe method of preparing PLO gels was developed to make it very easy to dispense the medication in unit dose syringes (Table 7-8). This method is extremely helpful when the individual dose of the medication is to be delivered in a tiny amount of the preparation. The preparation can easily and thoroughly be mixed between the **Luer lock (LL)** syringes and then loaded into oral syringes for easy, accurate dosing by the patient or caregiver.

TABLE 7-8 Syringe to Syringe Method for Preparing PLOs

Step 1	Calculate the required quantity of each ingredient for the total amount required on the MFR.
Step 2	Don appropriate PPE and clean the preparation area and equipment.
Step 3	Accurately weigh and/or measure each ingredient.
Step 4	Fill out the MCR and have the pharmacist check all calculations, ingredients, and volumes before mixing.
Step 5	Remove the plunger from one of the Luer lock (LL) syringes (Figure 7-2).
Step 6	Connect LL syringes using the LL to LL connector (Figure 7-3).
Step 7	Hold the connected syringes in a vertical orientation with the open syringe on top.
Step 8	Using the scaled measurements on the syringe, add the required amount of isopropyl palmitate/soy lecithin solution to the open syringe.
Step 9	Add active ingredient to the open syringe.
Step 10	If required in the MFR, add appropriate solvent (water, alcohol, propylene glycol, etc) to the open syringe.
Step 11	Using the scaled measurements on the syringe, add poloxamer gel to the open syringe to reach the required final volume (*QS AD*).
Step 12	Return the plunger to the open syringe. Flip the connected syringes. The syringe containing the preparation will now be on the bottom of the assembly.
Step 13	Disconnect the empty syringe (top) from the LL connector.
Step 14	*Carefully*, press on the plunger of syringe containing the preparation to remove the air captured when the plunger was replaced. Stop when the preparation can be seen moving into the LL connector.
Step 15	Reconnect the empty syringe to the LL connector.
Step 16	Pass the mixture back and forth between the syringes until homogeneous.
Step 17	Note: Poloxamer gel becomes thick as it warms. For thorough mixing, hold the bottom syringe with both hands and press the plunger against the counter to move the material into the top syringe.
Step 18	Flip and repeat per the MFR instructions.
Step 19	After the mixing is complete, push the entire product into 1 syringe and disconnect it from the LL to LL connector and empty syringe.
Step 20	Attach an "Luer lock to oral slip" (LL to OS) connector to the syringe containing the preparation (Figure 7-4).
Step 21	Insert the dispensing end of the oral syringe into the OS side of the connector (Figure 7-5).
Step 21	Holding the oral syringe in place, press the plunger of the LL syringe to move the preparation into the oral syringe to provide a unit dose.
Step 23	Repeat steps 1-19 until the required number of dispensing syringes has been filled.
Step 24	Label appropriately for dispensing.
Step 25	Get a final check by the pharmacist and finish filling out the MCR.

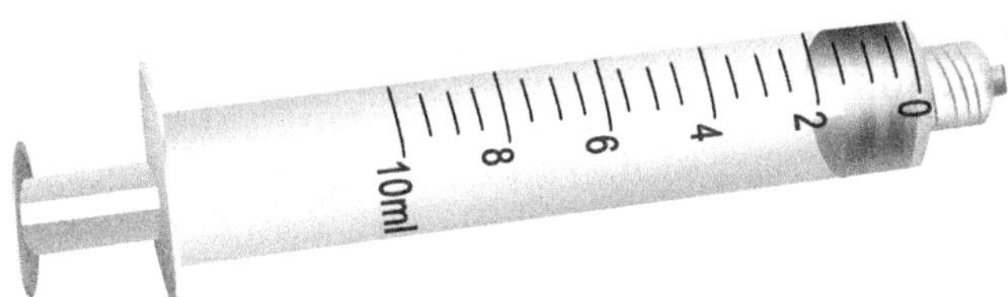

FIGURE 7-2 Luer lock syringe.

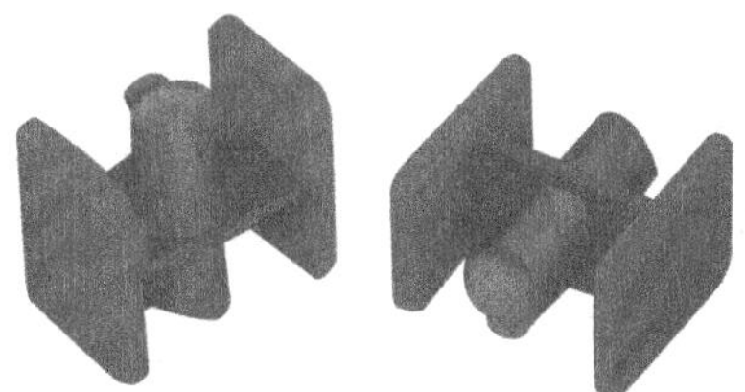

FIGURE 7-3 Luer to Luer connector.

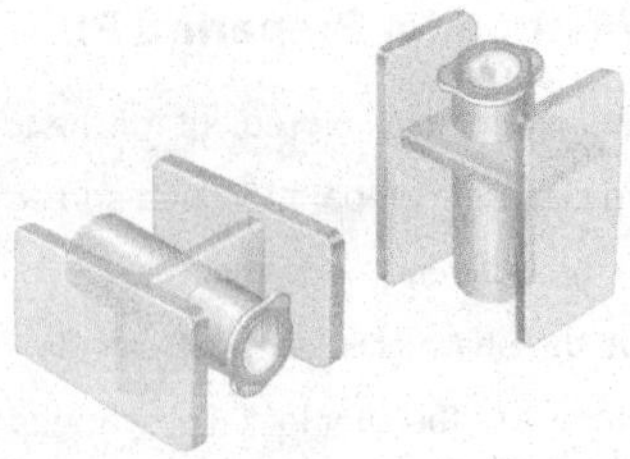

FIGURE 7-4 Luer lock to oral slip connector.

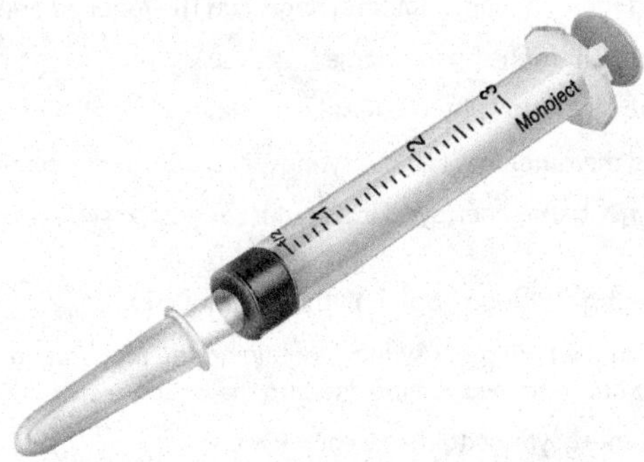

FIGURE 7-5 Oral syringe.

Educating patient on how to use this method for proper application to the skin should be part of the dispensing procedure to prevent the medication from being taken by mouth.

Metered Oval Pump Dispenser

Metered pump dispensers are composed of a cylinder with a vacuum mechanism in the top that is used to pump cream out of a container. The cylinders are loaded with a spatula, and when the base and lid are attached, an airtight seal is created. The button or lever on the top of the device is depressed several times to "prime" the pump by removing the air from the cylinder creating a vacuum. Then with each depression of the button or lever on the top of the device, the cream is dispensed (Figure 7-6).

Exact-Dose

The exact-dose dispenser is an attachment used with the specialized EMP jars discussed earlier in this chapter. The exact-dose has a large, easy-to-manipulate "key" that turns a mechanical ball and chamber mechanism. The device screws on to the threaded nipple on the lid of the jar (the threads used to attach the jar to the EMP for mixing). The patient turns the key to the vertical position to line the chamber up with the opening in the lid. The patient then pushes up on the bottom of the jar to fill the chamber with the preparation. As the cream moves into the chamber, it pushes the ball that moves toward the opening on the device and stops the cream from leaving the chamber. Now a measured amount of 0.5 g of the preparation is inside the chamber. Next, the patient turns the key 180 degrees so that the ball is next to the opening of the jar. The patient pushes on the bottom of the jar again, and the next dose of the preparation fills the chamber, pushes the ball to keep it from leaving the device, and also pushes the first dose out of the opening for application to the skin. The exact-dose is sturdy, easy to manipulate, and delivers an accurate, metered dose every time (Figure 7-7).

Topi-CLICK

Precise doses of semisolid medication compounds can also be measured accurately when dispensed in the Topi-CLICK dispenser. This device uses a screw mechanism to cause the cream to rise in the cylinder and come out the top. When the base of the device is turned, it clicks to indicate that a 0.25 g dose of the preparation has been pressed out through the opening on the top. The patient can hear the click and feel the device stop so they know they have dispensed an accurate dose (Figure 7-8).

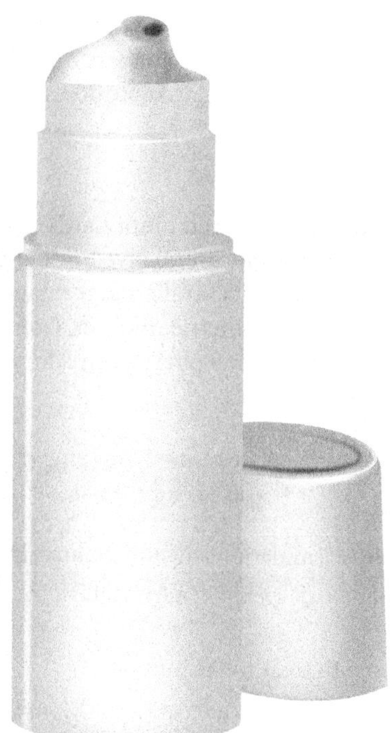

FIGURE 7-6 Metered oval pump dispensing device.

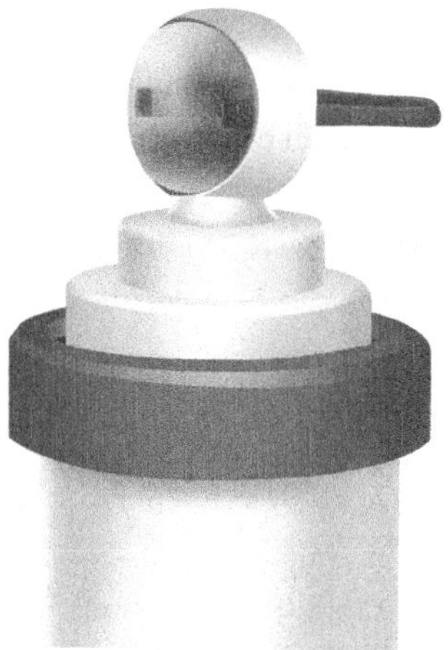

FIGURE 7-7 Exact-dose. (*Reproduced with permission from Unguator Technology.*)

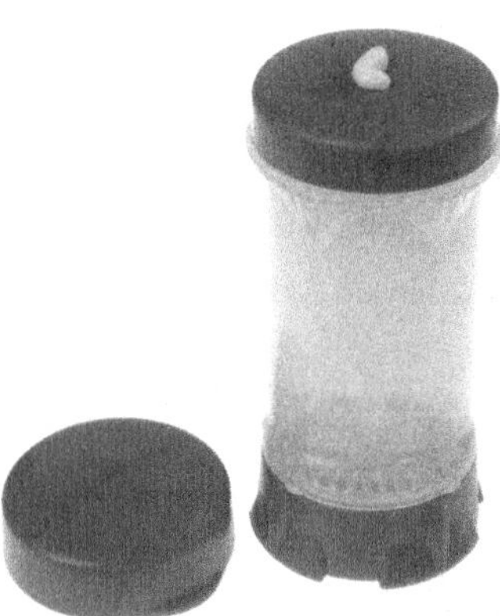

FIGURE 7-8 Topi-CLICK dispensing system. (*Reproduced with permission from Custom Rx TDA, LLC.*)

These devices are demonstrated at various sites on the Internet.

Using these devices instead of traditional tubes and jars can improve patient outcomes and quality of care because these devices provide more accurate doses of topical and TD formulations.

CONCLUSION

Simple compounded creams, ointments, gels, and lotions are common in the vast majority of compounding pharmacy practices. A technician involved in the preparation of this popular dosage form must know how to calculate concentration percentages accurately, as well as triturate powders and mix ingredients using geometric dilution. Compounding semisolid dosage forms is an important and valuable skill for any pharmacy technician.

CHAPTER SUMMARY

- The most common semisolid formulations include creams, lotions, gels, and ointments.
- Active medication ingredients are delivered in a semisolid formulation either transdermally or topically.
- Topical medications are used to treat the skin.
- Transdermal medications are used to deliver the drug past the skin into the bloodstream, muscle, or tissue.
- All calculations, APIs, solvents, and vehicles must be checked by the pharmacist before any compounding begins.
- Most active drug ingredients incorporated into a topical formulation should be able to dissolve into the vehicle.
- APIs are often suspended in transdermal formulations and ointments.
- The correct vehicle is chosen based on how the drug is to be delivered.
- A stabilized mixture of oil and water that does not separate is called an *emulsion*.
- Creams can be *water-in-oil* or *oil-in-water* emulsions.
- Most drugs and common solvents can be incorporated into one or the other type of emulsion.
- Lotions are thin versions of cream.
- Ointments are occlusive and do not contain water.
- Poloxamer gels were created as the vehicle for PLO gel, the original transdermal compounding vehicle.
- The 2 main sources for the drugs for topical and transdermal medications are prepared dosage forms and API powders.
- The EMP and the ointment mill are devices used for preparing semisolid dosage forms.
- A variety of precise dispensing devices are available to ensure proper dosing.
- PLO gel is commonly dispensed in oral syringes.

PTCB Review Questions

1. Which of the following statements are *true*?
   A. PLO gel is commonly dispensed in zip-lock bags.
   B. Ointments contain water.
   C. Topical medications are used to treat the skin.
   D. Never use geometric dilution when compounding semisolid formulations.
2. Common solvents used in compounding semisolid formulations include:
   A. Water, oil, and API
   B. Water, alcohol, and oil
   C. PLO gel and cream
   D. Ointment

3. Which of the following vehicles do not have occlusive properties?
   A. Petrolatum, White NF
   B. Poloxamer gel
   C. Lotion
   D. Ointment
4. Which manual steps in the mixing process may be skipped when using an EMP?
   A. Particle reduction
   B. Geometric dilution
   C. Levigation
   D. All of the above
5. What is an emulsion?
   A. A stabilized mixture of oil and water.
   B. An ointment.
   C. A semisolid dispensing device.
   D. None of the above.
6. Which of the following statements are *true*?
   A. The correct vehicle is chosen based on how the drug is to be delivered.
   B. A variety of precise dispensing devices are available to ensure proper dosing.
   C. All calculations, APIs, solvents, and vehicles do not need to be checked by the pharmacist.
   D. Both A and B.
7. What was the original transdermal compounding vehicle?
   A. Carbomer gel
   B. PLO gel
   C. Hydrophilic ointment
   D. Anhydrous gel
8. Which of the following is a main source of drug for topical and transdermal medications?
   A. Prepared dosage forms (tablets and capsules)
   B. Petrolatum, White NF
   C. Water and alcohol
   D. Both B and C
9. Which of the follow statements are *true*?
   A. Poloxamer gel thins as it warms.
   B. Carbomer gel thickens as it warms.
   C. Poloxamer gel thickens as it warms.
   D. Anhydrous gel thins as it warms.
10. How is a transdermal medication delivered to the bloodstream or tissue beneath the skin?
   A. By inhalation
   B. In a capsule
   C. Via liposomes on the skin
   D. In water or alcohol

Techs in Practice: Discussion Topics and Questions

SCENARIO 1

Research the development of transdermal medication delivery.

1. Who developed it?
2. When was it developed?
3. Explain the importance of the delivery system and its future implications for medicine.

SCENARIO 2

Technology is impacting every area of health care.
Use the Internet to find 2 innovative devices or technologies that are being used in compounding semisolid formulations.

Lab 1

Prepare the following formulation.
Give the product a correct BUD based on USP/NF Chapter ⟨795⟩ guidelines (see Chapter 4, Table 4-2).

Formulation	Baby Butt Cream	Total Quantity
		200 g

Equipment	
Electronic balance	
Mortar and pestle	
Compounding slab (tile)	
Graduated cylinder	
Rubber or metal spatula	
Ointment jar	
Ingredients	**Quantity**
Corn starch	60 g
Liquid antacid	72 mL
Menthol gel	6 g
White petrolatum	200 g

1. Perform any necessary calculations.
2. Gather supplies and measure ingredients.
3. Get pharmacist check.
4. Using mortar and pestle, triturate the corn starch to a fine powder.
5. Using geometric dilution, combine ingredients.
6. Place product in ointment jar and label appropriately.

Shelf life (BUD):

Quality assurance parameters	1. Total volume of 200 g 2. No visual particles 3. Product is smooth to the touch no grittiness

Lab 2

Using common references, list the APIs in the calculation exercises that are water soluble.

Calculation Review Questions

Calculate the amounts of each active ingredient that must be weighed/measured to complete the compounded preparations in questions 1, 2, and 3.

1. Ketoprofen 20%, cyclobenzaprine 2%, baclofen 2% in TD cream
   Calculate to make 120 g
2. Benzocaine 20%, lidocaine 6%, tetracaine 4% in topical cream
   Calculate to make 30 g
3. Ketamine 10%, amitriptyline 2% in TD Cream
   Calculate to make 60 g
4. Hydrocortisone 1% 120 g is prescribed. This preparation will use 2 ingredients: a manufactured hydrocortisone cream and a water-washable vehicle. The pharmacy has hydrocortisone 2.5% cream on hand. How many grams of hydrocortisone 2.5% cream and how much of the water-washable base are needed to fill this prescription?

This chapter includes the following PTCE Blueprint Knowledge Areas
Section 1.0-1.4 Strengths/dose, dosage forms, physical appearance, routes of administration, and duration of drug therapy.
Section 2.0-2.6 Record keeping, documentation, and retention (eg, length of time prescriptions are maintained on file).

Section 2.0-2.11 Infection control standards (eg, laminar air flow, clean room, hand washing, cleaning counting trays, countertop, and equipment). (OSHA, USP/NF Chapter ⟨795⟩ and ⟨797⟩)

Section 2.0-2.13 Professional standards regarding the roles and responsibilities of pharmacist, pharmacy technicians, and other pharmacy employees. (TJC, BOP)

Section 2.0-2.15 Facility, equipment, and supply requirements (eg, space requirements, prescription file storage, cleanliness, reference materials). (TJC, USP, BOP)

Section 3.0-3.3 Documentation (eg, batch preparation, compounding record).

Section 3.0-3.5 Selection and use of equipment and supplies.

Section 3.0-3.7 Non-sterile compounding processes.

Section 6.0-6.3 Calculate dosing required.

Section 6.0-6.4 Fill process (eg, select appropriate product, apply special handling requirements, and measure and prepare product for final check).

Section 6.0-6.5 Labeling requirements (eg, auxiliary and warning labels, expiration date, patient specific information).

Section 6.0-6.7 Dispensing process (eg, validation, documentation, and distribution).

Section 7.0-7.4 Storage requirements (eg, refrigeration, freezer, warmer).

This chapter includes the following Ex-CPT Test Specifications

Section 1 A-4 Comply with rules and regulations when filling prescriptions.

Section 1 A-6 Maintain a clean work environment in the pharmacy and patient care areas.

Section 1 C-7 Properly package prescription medication in child-resistant containers or other approved containers as required.

Section 1 C-8 Comply with professional, state, and federal laws and regulations.

Section 1 C-9 Use information found on medication stock bottles, such as drug name and strength, expiration date, and lot number.

Section 2 A-2 Differentiate among various dosage forms (eg, tablets vs capsules, ointment vs creams, and controlled release vs immediate release, parenteral vs oral).

Section 2 B-1 Interpret basic medical terminology commonly used in the pharmacy in order to effectively assist the pharmacist.

Section 3-B-2 Identify drugs that require special handling procedures.

Section 3 B-5 Follow proper record keeping procedures pertaining to the pharmacy.

Section 3 B-6 Follow the pharmacy's quality assurance policies and procedures.

Section 3 B-14 Properly and accurately prepare prescription labels.

Section 3 B-18 Use auxiliary labels properly.

Section 3 B-19 Properly label drug products packaged in approved containers or, when appropriate, original packages.

Section 3 C-2 Calculate the quantities of prescription medications to be dispensed.

Section 3 C-4 Properly calculate individual and daily dosages.

Section 3 D-1 Follow proper compounding procedures for non-sterile products.

Section 3 D-3 Properly repackage and label unit of use products.

Section 3 D-4 Properly calculate expiration dates for repackaged products.

This chapter includes the following ASHP Model Curriculum for Pharmacy Technician Training Goal Statements, Objectives, and Instructional Objectives

OBJ 3.3 Follow established laws and protocols to select the appropriate product.

OBJ 3.5 Accurately count or measure finished dosage forms as specified by the prescription medication order.

OBJ 3.6 Collect the correct ingredients for sterile or non-sterile products that require compounding.

OBJ 3.7 Accurately determine the correct amounts of ingredients for a compounded product.

OBJ 3.11 Follow safety policies and procedures in the preparation of all medications.

OBJ 3.13 Package the product in the appropriate type and size of container, using a manual process or automated system.

OBJ 3.14 Follow an established manual procedure or electronic procedure to generate accurate and complete product labels.

OBJ 3.18 Follow established policies and procedures for recording the preparation of bulk, unit dose, and special doses of medications prepared for immediate or in anticipation of future use.

OBJ 3.19 Follow the manufacturer's recommendation and/or the pharmacy's guidelines for storage of all medications prior to distribution.

OBJ 12.1 Follow policies and procedures for sanitation management, hazardous waste handling, and infection control.

OBJ 12.3 Maintain a clean and neat work environment.

OBJ 35.1 Apply the principles of quality assurance to all technician activities.

Answers to PTCB Questions

1. **C**
2. **B**
3. **C**
4. **D**
5. **A**
6. **D**
7. **B**
8. **A**
9. **C**
10. **C**

Answers to Calculation Questions

1. Ketoprofen 20% = 24 g
   Cyclobenzaprine 2% = 2.4 g
   Baclofen 2% = 2.4 g
2. Benzocaine 20% = 6 g
   Lidocaine 6% = 1.8 g
   Tetracaine 4% = 1.2 g
3. Ketamine 10% = 6 g
   Amitriptyline 2% = 1.2 g
4. Hydrocortisone 2.5% = 48 g
   Water-washable base = 72 g

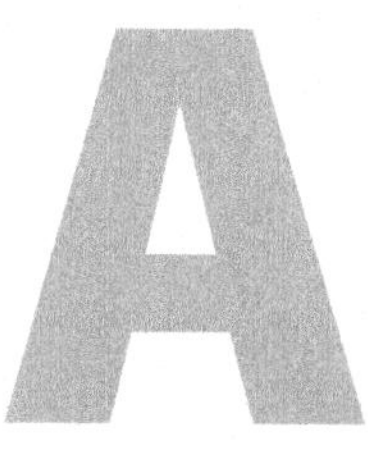

Common Abbreviations

Abbreviation	Meaning	Possible Confusion
a.c.	before meals	
a.d.	right ear	"a" can be mistaken as an "o" which could read "od," meaning right eye
AM	morning, before noon	
amp	ampule	
amt	amount	
aq	water	
API	active pharmaceutical ingredient	
a.s.	left ear	"a" can be mistaken as an "o" which could read "os"
ASA	aspirin	
ATC	around the clock	
au	both ears	"a" can be mistaken as an "o" which could read "ou," meaning both eyes
bid	twice daily	
BM	bowel movement	
BS	blood sugar	
BSA	body surface areas	
BUD	beyond-use date/dating (shelf life)	
cap, caps	capsule	
c	with (usually written with a bar on top of the "c")	
cc	cubic centimeter	mistaken for "U" also has an ambiguous meaning; use "mL" or "milliliters"
cmpd	compound	
cr, crm	cream	
D_5W	dextrose 5% solution	
D_5NS	dextrose 5% in normal saline (0.9%)	
DAW	dispense as written (ie, no generic substitution)	
dc, D/C, disc	discontinue or discharge	ambiguous meaning
DW	distilled water	
dx	diagnosis	
elix	elixir	
g	gram	

Abbreviation	Meaning	Possible Confusion
gr	grain	
gtt(s)	drop(s)	
h	hour	
hs	at bedtime or half-strength	ambiguous meaning
ID	intradermal	
IJ, inj	injection	mistaken for "IV"
IM	intramuscular	
IN	intranasal	mistaken for "IM" or "IV"
IP	intraperitoneal	
IU	international unit	mistaken for "IV" or "10," spell out "international unit"
IV	intravenous	
IVP	intravenous push	
IVPB	intravenous piggyback	
kg	kilogram	
KCl	potassium chloride	
liq	liquid	
LL	Luer lock	
lot	lotion	
M&P	mortar and pestle	
mcg	microgram	may be confused with "mg"
MCR	master compounding record	
MDF	manufactured drug formulation	
mEq	milliequivalent	
MFR	master formulation record	
mg	milligram	
$MgSO_4$	magnesium sulfate	may be confused with "MSO_4"
MMW	magic mouthwash	
mL	milliliter	
MS	morphine sulfate or magnesium sulfate	can mean either morphine sulfate or magnesium sulfate
MSO_4	morphine sulfate	may be confused with "$MgSO_4$"
MSDS	material safety data sheet	
NKA	no known allergies	
NKDA	no known drug allergies	
NPO	nothing by mouth	
NS	normal saline (0.9%)	
1/2NS	half normal saline (0.45%)	
od	right eye	"o" can be mistaken as an "a" which could read "a.d.," meaning right ear
os	left eye	"o" can be mistaken as an "a" which could read "a.s.," meaning left ear
ou	both eyes	"o" can be mistaken as an "a" which could read "au," meaning both ears
oz	ounce	
pc	after meals	
PEG	polyethylene glycol	
PM	evening or afternoon	
po	by mouth or orally	

Abbreviation	Meaning	Possible Confusion
pr	by rectum	
PRN, prn	as needed	
PV	via the vagina	
q	every, per	
qAM	every morning	
qPM	every afternoon/evening	
qhs.	every night at bedtime	
q1h	every 1 hour; (can replace "1" with other numbers)	
qd	every day	mistaken for "QOD"
qid	4 times a day	
q4PM	every day at 4 PM	mistaken to mean every 4 hours
qod	every other day	mistaken for "QD," spell out "every other day"
qqh	every 4 hours	
QS	a sufficient quantity	
QS AD	quantity sufficient to reach volume	
QWK	every week	
R	rectal	
RDT	rapid dissolving tablet	
SC, subc, subcut, subq, SQ	subcutaneous	"SC" can be mistaken for "SL," meaning sublingual
sig	directions	
SL	sublingually, under the tongue	
sol	solution	
ss	one-half or sliding scale	
stat	immediately	
supp	suppository	
susp	suspension	
sx	symptoms	
syr	syrup	
tab	tablet	
TT	tablet triturate	
TDD	transdermal drug delivery	
tbsp	tablespoon	
tid	3 times a day	
tiw	3 times a week	mistaken for twice a week
top	topical	
TPN	total parenteral nutrition	
tsp	teaspoon	
tx	treatment	
U	unit	mistaken for a "4," "0," or "cc"
μg	microgram	mistaken for "mg"
ud, ut dict	as directed	
ung	ointment	
vag	vaginally	
w/o	without	
YO	years old	

APPENDIX

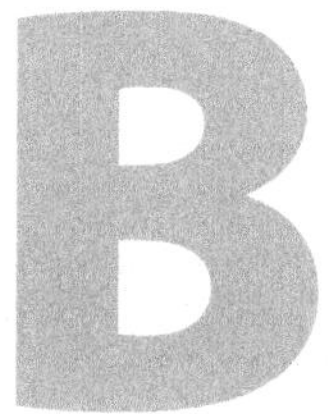

Student Competencies

PROPER USE OF ELECTRONIC BALANCE

Student Name: ________________________________ Date: ________________

Procedure		
Used appropriate hand washing techniques before compounding	YES	NO
Wore appropriate PPE for task being completed	YES	NO
Cleaned compounding area and equipment appropriately before compounding	YES	NO
Able to identify location of the MSDS, eye wash station, first-aid kit, and fire extinguisher	YES	NO
Gathered the proper supplies needed	YES	NO
Gathered the correct ingredients, the correct strengths	YES	NO
Properly performed any need calculations for ingredients	YES	NO
Checked that balance is leveled and at zero before using	YES	NO
Checked calibration log to make sure that balance had been calibrated	YES	NO
Tared balance after weigh boat/canoe/paper added	YES	NO
Weighed each ingredient separately and placed powder with original container	YES	NO
Tared scale between each ingredient weighed	YES	NO
Asked for a final check of each weighed ingredient	YES	NO
Cleaned up work area and equipment after compounding is completed	YES	NO
Instructor Comments:		

By signing below, I certify this student has demonstrated 100% competency at the tasks above.

Instructor name ________________________________ Date________________

Instructor signature ________________________________

FILLING CAPSULES USING THE "PUNCH" METHOD (SOLID FORMULATION)

Student Name: ____________________________ Date: ____________

Procedure		
Used appropriate hand washing techniques before compounding	YES	NO
Wore appropriate PPE for task being completed	YES	NO
Cleaned compounding area and equipment appropriately before compounding	YES	NO
Able to identify location of the MSDS, eye wash station, first-aid kit, and fire extinguisher	YES	NO
Gathered the proper supplies needed to compound as documented in MFR	YES	NO
Gathered the correct ingredients, the correct strengths	YES	NO
Properly performed any need calculations for ingredients	YES	NO
Measured proper amounts of each ingredient including extra to account for loss	YES	NO
Documented necessary information on MCR and asked for a check before beginning compounding	YES	NO
Properly used geometric dilution to combine ingredients	YES	NO
Arranged combined ingredients properly on ointment slab/paper	YES	NO
Properly separated capsules	YES	NO
Properly filled capsules using "punch" method	YES	NO
Replaced capsule caps and weighed each capsule	YES	NO
Added or removed powder to achieve correct weight	YES	NO
Used all powders	YES	NO
Properly "locked capsules"	YES	NO
Completed all documentation for finished product on MCR	YES	NO
Removed excess powders from capsules	YES	NO
Properly packaged finished capsules	YES	NO
Properly labeled finish product including correct BUD (shelf life)	YES	NO
Asked for a final check	YES	NO
Cleaned up work area and equipment after compounding is completed	YES	NO
Instructor Comments:		

By signing below, I certify this student has demonstrated 100% competency at the tasks above.

Instructor name ____________________________ Date______________

Instructor signature________________________________

PREPARATION OF A COMPOUNDED ORAL LIQUID SUSPENSION

Student Name: ______________________________ Date: ____________

Procedure		
Used appropriate hand washing techniques before compounding	YES	NO
Wore appropriate PPE for task being completed	YES	NO
Cleaned compounding area and equipment appropriately before compounding	YES	NO
Able to identify location of the MSDS, eye wash station, first-aid kit, and fire extinguisher	YES	NO
Gathered the proper supplies needed to compound as documented in MFR	YES	NO
Gathered the correct ingredients, the correct strengths	YES	NO
Properly performed any need calculations for ingredients	YES	NO
Documented necessary information on MCR and asked for a check before beginning compounding	YES	NO
Triturated tablets or powders to uniform-sized particles	YES	NO
Properly used "geometric dilution" to combine powder and vehicle	YES	NO
Poured combined products into a proper container (beaker, graduated cylinder)	YES	NO
Rinsed remaining particles from M&P with vehicle	YES	NO
Properly added vehicle to achieve final volume (QS AD)	YES	NO
Properly packaged finished product	YES	NO
Properly labeled finished product including BUD (shelf life) and auxiliary labels	YES	NO
Completed all documentation for finished product on MCR	YES	NO
Asked for a final check	YES	NO
Cleaned up work area after compounding is completed	YES	NO
Instructor Comments:		

By signing below, I certify this student has demonstrated 100% competency at the tasks above.

Instructor name ______________________________ Date____________

Instructor signature ______________________________

SEMISOLID FORMULATION

Student Name: ______________________________ Date: ______________

Procedure		
Used appropriate hand washing techniques before compounding	YES	NO
Wore appropriate PPE for task being completed	YES	NO
Cleaned compounding area and equipment appropriately before compounding	YES	NO
Able to identify location of the MSDS, eye wash station, first-aid kit, and fire extinguisher	YES	NO
Gathered the proper supplies needed to compound as documented in MFR	YES	NO
Gathered the correct ingredients, the correct strengths	YES	NO
Properly performed any need calculations for ingredients	YES	NO
Measured proper amounts of each ingredient	YES	NO
Documented necessary information on MCR and asked for a check before beginning compounding	YES	NO
Triturated (active) powdered ingredients to uniform particle size	YES	NO
Added proper solvent to each powder	YES	NO
Combined with appropriate vehicle as instructed on MFR using geometric dilution	YES	NO
Performed quality assurance checks as instructed in MFR	YES	NO
Properly packaged finished product	YES	NO
Properly labeled finished product including BUD (shelf life)	YES	NO
Completed all documentation for finished product on MCR	YES	NO
Asked for a final check	YES	NO
Cleaned up work area and equipment after compounding is completed	YES	NO
Instructor Comments:		

By signing below, I certify this student has demonstrated 100% competency at the tasks above.

Instructor name ______________________________ Date______________

Instructor signature ______________________________

APPENDIX C

Practice Formulations

Lab 1

ASPIRIN SUPPOSITORY: 325 mg

Calculated to make 12: suppositories

Ingredients

Aspirin powder	3.9 G
Peg blend	22.5 G
OR	
Fatty acid suppository base	17.94 G

Supplies

Balance
Weigh papers, boats, canoes, etc
Hot plate
Beaker
Disposable/dispensable suppository molds
Mortar and pestle

Procedure

1 Calculate the required quantity of each ingredient for the total amount to be prepared
2 Accurately weigh and/or measure each ingredient
3 Melt suppository base to 55°–60°C
4 Reduce aspirin particles to uniform size using mortar and pestle
5 Sprinkle aspirin into melted suppository base while stirring
6 Pour mixture into disposable suppository molds
7 Cool at room temperature
8 Package and dispense

Storage Instructions

Store finished suppositories in refrigerator.

Beyond-use Date

The earliest expiration date of any ingredient or 6 months from date prepared (whichever comes first).

For instructional use only

Lab 2

Drug Name	Route	Dosage Form	Concentration
Lip Balm	Topical	Medication Stick	5:3

Equipment
- Beaker
- Hot plate
- Weigh boat
- Beaker tongs
- Medication stick
- Mortar and pestle
- Stirring rod
- Metal spatula
- Electronic balance

Ingredients	Quantity (g)
Cocoa Butter 5 g	5
Petrolatum White NF	3

Compounding Procedures

1. Perform necessary calculations
2. Weigh ingredients
3. Triturate the Cocoa Butter into a fine powder in mortar
4. Melt Cocoa Butter in a beaker, constantly stirring
5. Add white petrolatum and mix thoroughly (do not burn mixture)
6. Let mixture cool slightly (cool to the back of the hand)
7. Pour an even amount of mixture into 2 medication sticks
8. Let cool until hardened at room temperature
9. Label appropriately

Beyond-use Date: The earliest expiration date of any ingredient or 6 months from date prepared (whichever comes first).

Formula Quantity: 2 sticks

Auxiliary Labels/Storage: External use only, store at room temperature

For instructional use only

Lab 3

Drug Name	Route	Dosage Form	Concentration
Progesterone Soft Troches	Oral	Troche	100 mg/1 g Troche

Equipment
- Hot plate
- 100-mL beaker
- Sieve
- Disposable troche mold
- Electronic balance
- Stir rod
- Mortar and pestle
- Spatula

Ingredients	Quantity
Progesterone (wettable)	3 g
Polyethylene glycol 1450	28 g
Sucrose	2 g
Mint extract	2-3 gtt

Compounding Procedures

1. Perform any necessary calculations
2. Weigh progesterone
3. Mix progesterone and sugar by geometric dilution and trituration
4. Melt the PEG 1450 into a 100-mL beaker stirring thoroughly
5. Sieve the powders through a mesh screen into the melted PEG
6. Ensure each addition is wetted before adding additional powder
7. Mix thoroughly
8. Remove beaker from heat, allow to cool slightly
9. Add mint extract and mix thoroughly
10. Pour mixture into troche mold, overfilling cavities
11. Let harden
12. Dispense in disposable mold and label appropriately

Beyond-use Date: The earliest expiration date of any ingredient or 6 months from date prepared (whichever comes first).

Formula Quantity: 30 Troches

Auxiliary Labels/Storage: Store at room temperature

For instructional use only

Lab 4

Thiamine 25 mg/mL Oral Suspension **Available Commercial Product: Thiamine 100 mg tablets** **Total Prepared Volume: 120 mL**	
Ingredients Thiamine 100 mg: 30 tablets Oral suspending vehicle: 60 mL Oral syrup vehicle: QS to 120 mL Strawberry syrup: 5 mL	
Equipment and Supplies Mortar and pestle Graduate	
Compounding Process	
Step 1	In an appropriate mortar and pestle, triturate tablets to a fine powder
Step 2	Add a small amount of oral suspending vehicle and levigate to form a paste
Step 3	Using geometric dilution, add remainder of oral suspending vehicle mixing thoroughly between each addition
Step 4	Transfer contents of the mortar to a graduated cylinder
Step 5	Rinse the mortar and pestle with strawberry syrup and pour into graduated cylinder
Step 6	QS to a total volume of 120 mL with oral syrup vehicle
Step 7	Transfer to 4 oz amber bottle and label appropriately
BUD/Storage	The earliest expiration date of any ingredient or 91 days (whichever comes first)/ room temperature or refrigerated.
References	*Intern J Pharm Compounding*. 2007;11(3):250.
Labeling	Thiamine oral suspension 25 mg/mL
Auxiliary Labels	Shake well
Quality Check	Powders should be evenly distributed
Notes	May substitute thiamine hydrochloride USP powder instead of thiamine tablets.

For instructional use only

Lab 5

Triamcinolone 0.025% in Water-Washable Base						
Manufacture	Lot #	EXP	Ingredients	Amounts	Prep initial's	Check initial's
			Triamcinolone acetonide powder	0.105 g		
			Water-washable base UMF	420 g		

Equipment	Device #
• Beaker	
• Electronic balance	
• Hot plate	
• Weigh boat or paper	
• Electric or hand mixer	
• Rubber spatula	
• Ceramic mixing bowl (large)	

Compounding Instructions

1. Weigh ingredients
2. Melt water-washable base in beaker
3. Combine powder and a portion of melted base in mixing bowl
4. Mix with rubber spatula until mixture is smooth
5. Transfer remaining melted base into mixing bowl
6. Mix formulation with hand mixer or electric mixer on low-speed until smooth and thick
7. Transfer to 1-lb ointment jar and label appropriately

Auxiliary Label	Beyond-use Date	
For external use only	The earliest expiration date of any ingredient or 6 months from date prepared. (whichever comes first)	Reference for formulation: ____________ Reference for BUD: ____________

Quality Assurance
- White cream
- Smooth and thick
- No visible particles

Total volume of prepared cream
420 g (maybe slightly more)

Labeling
Drug name______________
Strength______________
Amount prepared_________
Date prepped___________
Formulation lot #__________

Final check by: Label check by: Date checked:

For instructional use only

Lab 6

Magic Mouthwash						
Manufacture	Lot #	EXP	Ingredients	Amounts	Prep initial's	Check initial's
			Lidocaine viscous 2%	60 mL		
			Maalox or generic equivalent	60 mL		
			Diphenhydramine elixir (alcohol free) 12.5 mg/5 mL	60 mL		

Equipment	Device #
• 3 graduated cylinders	
• 4 or 6 oz amber bottle	

Compounding Instructions

1. Measure separate ingredients into 3 graduated cylinders
2. Pour all 3 ingredients into amber dispensing bottle
3. Shake well
4. Label appropriately

Auxiliary Label	Shelf Life (BUD)	
Shake well Swish and spit solution	14 days from date prepared or the earliest expiration date of any ingredient (whichever comes first)	Reference for formulation: ________________ Reference for BUD: ________________

Notes: Use original Maalox or GEQ—do not use Maalox plus

Labeling
Drug name_______________
Strength________________
Amount prepared__________
Date prepped____________
Formulation lot #____________

Final check by:	Label check by:	Date checked:

For instructional use only

APPENDIX

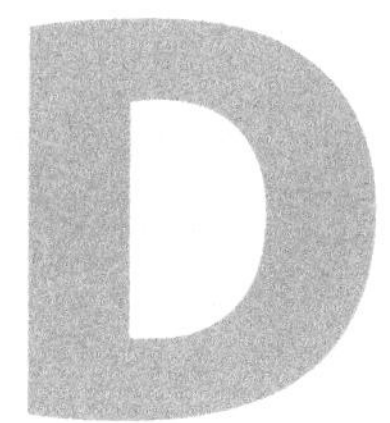

USP/NF Storage Conditions and Beyond Use Dating Parameters

Storage and Temperature Conditions	USP/NF Definition
Freezer	Temperature maintained at between −25° and −10°C
Refrigerator	Temperature maintained between 2° and 8°C
Cold	Any temperature not exceeding 8°C
Cool	Temperatures between 8° and 15°C
Room temperature	General temperature prevailing in a work environment
Controlled room temperature	Temperatures between 20° and 25°C
	Excursions are allowed between 15° and 30°C in pharmacies, hospitals, and warehouses
	Spikes up to 40°C are permitted for no more than 24 h
Warm	Temperature ranges between 30° and 40°C
Excessive heat	Any temperature between 30° and 40°C
Dry place	Does not exceed 40% humidity at 20°C
Protection from freezing	Freezing will cause a loss of potency or strength or a destructive alteration of properties to the product
Protection from light	Light will cause a loss of strength or potency or a destructive alteration of properties to the product

USP/NF Chapter ⟨795⟩ Beyond-use Dates for Non-sterile Compounded Formulations in the Absence of Stability Data

Formulation	Beyond-use Dates
Oral formulations prepared in **aqueous** vehicles	14 days, under refrigeration or the earliest expiration date of any component in the formulation, whichever comes first.
Nonaqueous formulations	Maximum of 6 months or the earliest expiration date of any component in the formulation, whichever comes first.
Aqueous topical and **semisolid** formulations	Maximum of 30 days or the earliest expiration date of any component in the formulation, whichever comes first.
Solid dosage forms	The earliest expiration date of any component in the formulation, or a maximum of 6 months, whichever comes first.

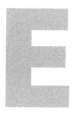

APPENDIX

Final Exam

1. Compounding accounts for what percentage of prescribed medication in the United States?
   A. 5%
   B. 50%
   C. 1%
   D. 3%
2. In what year was USP/NF first published?
   A. 1920
   B. 1875
   C. 1820
   D. None of the above
3. Which of the following would allow for a pharmacy to compound a medication for a patient?
   A. The patient requires a different concentration of the active drug than can be provided by a manufactured medication.
   B. The doctor wants to save the patient money.
   C. The manufactured product available contains an ingredient that the patient cannot tolerate.
   D. Both A and C.
4. The rules for nonsterile pharmacy compounding are established in which chapter of the USP/NF?
   A. Chapter ⟨795⟩
   B. Chapter ⟨797⟩
   C. Chapter ⟨597⟩
   D. Chapter ⟨595⟩
5. Which of the following statements are *true*?
   A. A compounding pharmacy must have a compounding certification from the PCAB in order to perform pharmacy compounding.
   B. The state board of pharmacy regulates pharmacy compounding in their specific state.
   C. Chapter ⟨797⟩ of the USP/NF defines all nonsterile compounding rules and regulations.
   D. Both A and C are true statements.
6. 8 g = ________mg
   A. 0.08
   B. 800
   C. 80
   D. 8000
7. 68 kg + 44 kg = ________lb
   A. 246.4
   B. 264.4
   C. 112
   D. 264
8. A child weighs 37.5 lb; the medication is prescribed to be given at 3.5 mg/kg twice daily. How many grams of medication will be given to the child each day?
   A. 11.9 g
   B. 0.119 g
   C. 1.19 g
   D. 119 g

9. 44 oz of a medication is dispensed to a patient who weighs 79.5 kg. How many total doses will the patient take if the prescription directions read: 20 mL 3 times daily?
   A. 22 doses
   B. 44 doses
   C. 79.5 doses
   D. 66 doses
10. 1 gal of 0.45% sodium chloride = ____________ L
   A. 3840
   B. 3.84
   C. 384
   D. 0.39
11. 78°C = ________°F
   A. 25.6
   B. 127.4
   C. 256
   D. 172.4
12. A prescription is written for 45 g of hydrocortisone 7.5% in water-washable base. The pharmacy has hydrocortisone 20%. How much hydrocortisone 20% is needed to fill this prescription?
   A. 28.1 g
   B. 20 g
   C. 16.9 g
   D. 1.69 g
13. Benzocaine 12%, tetracaine 2%, lidocaine 3% in topical cream. How much of each ingredient is needed to prepare 60 g?
   A. Benzocaine 1.2 g, tetracaine 7.2 g, lidocaine 1.8 g
   B. Benzocaine 1.8 g, tetracaine 7.2 g, lidocaine 1.2 g
   C. Benzocaine 7.2 g, tetracaine 1.2 g, lidocaine 1.8 g
   D. Benzocaine 1.2 g, tetracaine 1.8 g, lidocaine 7.2 g
14. Ketoprofen 12%, cyclobenzaprine 1%, baclofen 5% in 160 g of a transdermal cream. How much ketoprofen is required for this formulation?
   A. 1.92 g
   B. 192 g
   C. 92 g
   D. 19.2 g
15. A patient weighing 122 lb is to take 3 mg/kg of a medication twice a day for 14 days. The medication comes 5 mg/mL. How much medication will be needed to complete the 14-day regimen?
   A. 932.4 mL
   B. 93.4 mL
   C. 55.5 mL
   D. 955.5 mL
16. What auxiliary label must be attached to a compounded oral liquid suspension?
   A. For external use only
   B. Do not crush or chew
   C. Shake well
   D. None of the above
17. Which reference provides guidance in assigning a Beyond-use date (BUD) to a nonsterile compounded preparation?
   A. USP/NF Chapter ⟨797⟩
   B. USP/NF Chapter ⟨795⟩
   C. *Trissel's Stability of Compounded Formulations*
   D. Both B and C
18. Which capsule size has a largest capacity?
   A. 2
   B. 000
   C. 00
   D. 4

19. In what document would you find toxicity and safety information about a substance or chemical used in a sterile compound?
    A. MFR
    B. MSDS
    C. SOP
    D. MCR
20. What piece of compounding equipment has a powerful motor and 3 ceramic rollers?
    A. Electronic mortar and pestle
    B. Powder hood
    C. Both A and B
    D. Ointment mill
21. How many grams of drug are in 240 mL of a 12% solution?
    A. 28.8 g
    B. 288 g
    C. 2880 g
    D. 2.88 g
22. Which of the following statements are *true*?
    A. A gram is a smaller unit of measure than a milligram.
    B. 1 mL is equal to 1 oz
    C. One tablespoon is equal to 15 mL
    D. 1 mL is larger than 1 L
23. Which of the following is a mixture of a powder and liquid in which the powder completely dissolves into the liquid?
    A. Solvent
    B. Solute
    C. Suspension
    D. Solution
24. How many grams are equal to 16 oz?
    A. 454 g
    B. 2.2 kg
    C. 4.54 g
    D. Both B and C
25. 1 gal = __________ mL
    A. 4890 mL
    B. 3840 mL
    C. 3849 mL
    D. 48.9 mL
26. Which of the following compounded dosage forms contains 10% alcohol?
    A. Oil
    B. Preserved water
    C. Elixirs
    D. Starch
27. Which of the following statements are *true*?
    A. An enema is a liquid formulation administered to the vagina.
    B. Both C and D are true statements.
    C. An enema is a liquid formulation administered to the rectum.
    D. A douche is a liquid formulation administered to the vagina.
28. Which of the following are vehicles used in compounding liquid formulations?
    A. Petrolatum
    B. Water
    C. Structured suspending vehicles
    D. Both B and C
29. Which compounding vehicle is an effective growth media for all living things?
    A. Syrup
    B. Oil
    C. Polyethylene glycol
    D. Water

30. What is the smallest amount that can be accurately weighed on an analytical balance?
    A. 2 mg
    B. 20 mg
    C. 0.2 mg
    D. 20 g
31. Which piece of equipment will assist in preventing air and movement from affecting the accuracy of an electronic balance?
    A. Calibration weight
    B. Beaker
    C. Air shield
    D. Weigh canoes
32. 1 g of metronidazole is equal to 1.6 g of metronidazole benzoate. How much metronidazole benzoate must be weighed to provide 10 g of metronidazole?
    A. 1.6 g
    B. 16 g
    C. 160 g
    D. None of the above
33. Which of the following statements are *false*?
    A. A transdermal medication is delivered into the bloodstream, muscle, or tissue.
    B. A troche delivers medication by dissolving in the buccal cavity.
    C. A topical medication is delivered into the bloodstream, muscle, or tissue.
    D. A sublingual medication is delivered under the tongue through the mucous membrane.
34. Which of the following is a common semisolid compounded formulation?
    A. Gel
    B. Capsule
    C. Troche
    D. Oral suspension
35. Which piece of compounding equipment has specialized jars and a spinning mixing blade?
    A. Ointment mill
    B. Homogenizer
    C. Electronic mortar and pestle
    D. Hot plate
36. How are active medications delivered in semisolid formulations?
    A. Sublingually
    B. Topically
    C. Orally
    D. Both A and B
37. Which of the following is a synthetic wax produced in various molecular weights used in compounding?
    A. Cellulose
    B. Methylcellulose gel
    C. PEG
    D. Syrup
38. What is the most common excipient used in preparing capsules?
    A. Alum lake dye
    B. Gelatin
    C. Lactose monohydrate powder
    D. PEG
39. What is longest BUD a tablet triturate can be assigned if no other stability information exists?
    A. 14 days from the date prepared
    B. 3 months from the date prepared
    C. 30 days from the date prepared
    D. None of the above
40. Which are the 2 primary vehicles used in compounding suppositories?
    A. Bases that melt and bases that dissolve
    B. Hypromellose and water
    C. Structured suspension vehicles and distilled water
    D. Both B and C

41. What is the longest BUD that can be given to an aqueous oral liquid when there is no other stability information available?
    A. 30 days at controlled room temperature
    B. 14 days refrigerated
    C. 6 months at controlled room temperature
    D. 3 months at controlled room temperature
42. A lip balm is considered what type of formulation?
    A. Semisolid
    B. Solid
    C. Liquid
    D. Both A and C
43. Which of the following statements are *true*?
    A. Syrup contains 10% alcohol.
    B. Elixirs should always be administered topically.
    C. A suspension is a mixture of powder and liquid in which the powder is surrounded by liquid.
    D. A RDT is a considered a semisolid formulation.
44. 3:00 PM is the same as ______ in international/military time.
    A. 1500
    B. 0300
    C. 1400
    D. 1700
45. What information must be included in the MFR for a compounded formulation?
    A. The name of the physician that prescribed the medication.
    B. The patient's date of birth.
    C. Quality parameters for assessing the preparation before it is dispensed.
    D. All of the above.
46. What is the pharmacy definition of "QS AD"?
    A. Quality Sufficient to reach volume
    B. Triturate
    C. Crush to uniform particle size
    D. Quantity Sufficient to reach volume
47. What is the definition of hydrophilic?
    A. Thickened liquid
    B. Water loving
    C. Particles suspended in liquid
    D. Through the skin
48. A liquid medication is ordered at 3 mg/kg once daily for a patient who weighs 97 lb. The medication is compounded as a 5-mg/mL solution. How much medication is needed to provide a 7-day supply? Round the answer to the nearest tenth.
    A. 18.5 mL
    B. 1848 mL
    C. 185 mL
    D. 26 mL
49. USP/NF defines controlled room temperature as
    A. Temperature between 20° and 25°C
    B. Temperatures between 30° and 40°C
    C. Temperatures between 2° and 8°C
    D. Temperatures between 8° and 15°C
50. An ointment is considered which type of formulation?
    A. Liquid
    B. Semisolid
    C. Solid
    D. None of the above

APPENDIX

F Veterinary Compounding

Compounding medications for animals has been traditionally done in the veterinary clinic by the veterinarian himself, but the industry has grown substantially over recent years, and many veterinarian practices have given this task over to compounding pharmacies.

Pharmacies that compound medications for human consumption can also compound medications for animals. All the same rules of compounding that apply to human patients apply to animals, with the same goals of providing the exact dose needed in a form that achieves patient compliance and improves outcomes. Manufactured medications approved for veterinary use are available in dosage forms that fit normal veterinary dosing needs. However, veterinarians rely heavily on human medications in providing for their animal patients. For example, the human dose of a medication might be 1 tablet, but for a small dog or cat, the correct dose may be 1/5 of the tablet. The pharmacy could compound the correct dose of the medication in an oral liquid or a treat.

Veterinary compounding is a growing area of pharmacy. The compounding pharmacy interested in serving veterinary patients can find a great deal of information, articles, and formulations in the *International Journal of Pharmaceutical Compounding.*

A pharmacy technician with familiarity and knowledge related to this specialty area of practice can provide needed expertise and skills to a pharmacy that is moving forward into veterinary medicine.

Examples of Frequently Prescribed Medications, Dosage Forms, and Vehicles Used in Veterinary Compounding

Apomorphine tablet triturates: Used when an animal swallows something harmful	• Veterinarian will administer in the **office only** • Tablet is administered into the conjunctiva of the eye • Induces vomiting
Potassium bromide capsules: Used in conjunction with phenobarbital to control epilepsy	• Potassium bromide is not approved for any use in humans • No commercial tablet or capsule to use as source of drug • Can also be provided as an oral liquid
Oral liquids	• The same vehicles used for humans can be used for dogs • Veterinary flavorings are available (beef, chicken, liver, bacon, tuna and sardine, etc) • Methylcellulose 1% gel is often used to prepare oral liquids for feline patients
Veterinary chews	• Prepared using a troche mold • Pharmacies have developed their own formulations
PLO gel: Used as a vehicle to deliver select medications to cats	• Is rubbed into the pinna (the inside, hairless area) of the ear • Drug is intended to enter the bloodstream transdermally

Sample Veterinary Formulation

Veterinary chews 20 mg API treats

Ingredients

50 g: Ground moist (semi soft) animal treat
25 g: Gelatin vehicle
API

Equipment

Balance
Troche mold
Hot plate
Beaker
Spatula
Mortar and pestle

Preparation Instructions

1. Calculate and weigh/measure required amount of active ingredients.
2. Subtract weight of API from calculated weight of chosen treat.
3. Crush chosen treat into powder.
4. Incorporate API evenly into the crushed treat.
5. Melt gelatin vehicle.
6. Add to the powder and stir thoroughly until the combined ingredients have the consistency of moist cookie dough.
7. Spread into troche mold.
8. Let set until firm.
9. Package appropriately.

Note: Do not use treats with "cheese" centers.

Index

Note: Page numbers followed by *f* or *t* indicate figures or tables, respectively.

CPSIA information can be obtained
at www.ICGtesting.com
Printed in the USA
FSOW04n0408110717
36139FS

9 780071 829885